Certified Medical Assistant Exam Practice Questions

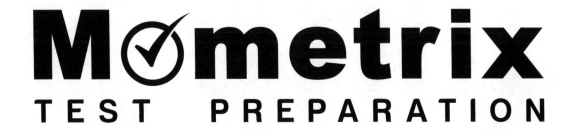

TEST PREPARATION

DEAR FUTURE EXAM SUCCESS STORY

First of all, **THANK YOU** for purchasing Mometrix study materials!

Second, congratulations! You are one of the few determined test-takers who are committed to doing whatever it takes to excel on your exam. **You have come to the right place.** We developed these practice tests with one goal in mind: to deliver you the best possible approximation of the questions you will see on test day.

Standardized testing is one of the biggest obstacles on your road to success, which only increases the importance of doing well in the high-pressure, high-stakes environment of test day. Your results on this test could have a significant impact on your future, and these practice tests will give you the repetitions you need to build your familiarity and confidence with the test content and format to help you achieve your full potential on test day.

Your success is our success

We would love to hear from you! If you would like to share the story of your exam success or if you have any questions or comments in regard to our products, please contact us at **800-673-8175** or **support@mometrix.com**.

Thanks again for your business and we wish you continued success!

Sincerely,
The Mometrix Test Preparation Team

TABLE OF CONTENTS

Practice Test #1

1. Which level of Maslow's theory of human behavior requires achievement, independence, and self-respect?

    a. Social.
    b. Esteem.
    c. Safety.
    d. Self-actualization.

2. Which of the following milestones would not be expected of a 4-month-old?

    a. The ability to coo.
    b. The ability to place objects in the mouth.
    c. The ability to roll from front to back.
    d. The ability to sit down without help.

3. Which of the following is a basic conflict for childhood ages newborn to 18 months according to Erikson's stages of psychosocial development?

    a. Initiative vs. guilt.
    b. Identity vs. role confusion.
    c. Autonomy vs. shame/doubt.
    d. Trust vs. mistrust.

4. Which of the following milestones would be expected of an 18-month-old?

    a. To be able to briefly balance and hop on one foot.
    b. To be able to use plurals and pronouns.
    c. To be able to use a spoon and cup with assistance.
    d. To have a vocabulary of several hundred words.

5. Which level of Maslow's theory of human behavior requires realizing one's personal potential?

    a. Safety.
    b. Physiological.
    c. Self-actualization.
    d. Social.

6. A person who throws a book at a wall during an argument and blames her partner for hostile behavior is displaying which type of defense mechanism?

    a. Projection.
    b. Regression.
    c. Compartmentalization.
    d. Acting out.

7. After being told that he has lung cancer, the patient offers to stop smoking immediately. He is in which stage of grief according to Kübler-Ross?

    a. Bargaining.
    b. Anger.
    c. Denial.
    d. Grief.

8. Which of the following is not an appropriate method of communication to someone who is hearing impaired?

    a. Hand gestures.
    b. Pantomiming.
    c. Speaking especially loudly.
    d. Drawing pictures.

9. Which of the following is an external barrier to communication?

    a. Weather.
    b. Pain.
    c. Hunger.
    d. Anger.

10. According to Erikson's psychosocial stages of development, when does the conflict identity vs. role confusion occur?

    a. Adolescence.
    b. Young adulthood.
    c. Middle adulthood.
    d. Young childhood.

11. Being able to relate personal experiences to a particular situation displays which of the following types of understanding?

    a. Reflection.
    b. Restatement.
    c. Clarification.
    d. Feedback.

12. Which of the following levels of Maslow's theory of human behavior need to be fulfilled first?

    a. Physiological.
    b. Safety.
    c. Social.
    d. Esteem.

13. A person who repeatedly loses track of time after experiencing a traumatic event is likely undergoing which form of denial?

    a. Rationalization.
    b. Disassociation.
    c. Denial.
    d. Displacement.

14. A patient is given the diagnosis of metastatic breast cancer and subsequently becomes sullen and solitary. She is in which stage of grief, according to Kübler-Ross?

    a. Denial.
    b. Grief.
    c. Acceptance.
    d. Depression.

15. According to Erikson's psychosocial stages of development, what basic conflict do children face in elementary school?

    a. Autonomy vs. shame/doubt.
    b. Intimacy vs. isolation.
    c. Industry vs. inferiority.
    d. Integrity vs. despair.

16. Which of the following nonverbal cues display anger?

    a. Hunched posture, remaining at a distance, limited eye contact.
    b. Touching frequently, low voice, sustained eye contact.
    c. Rigid posture, standing in close proximity, sudden movements/gestures.
    d. Standing in close proximity, slow purposeful gestures, relaxed posture.

17. Which of the following milestones would not be expected of a 5-year-old?

    a. Skips, jumps, and hops with good balance.
    b. Follow 5 commands in a row.
    c. Knows telephone number.
    d. Has a vocabulary of more than 2,000 words.

18. According to Erikson's psychosocial stages of development, which of the following people would be facing the conflict of initiative vs. guilt?

    a. 6-year-old.
    b. 16-year-old.
    c. 26-year-old.
    d. 36-year-old.

19. A patient who is chronically homeless may have difficulties effectively communicating because of which of the following internal barriers?

    a. Anger.
    b. Pain.
    c. Hunger.
    d. Sadness.

20. At what age would the average baby begin to crawl?

    a. 3 months.
    b. 9 months.
    c. 18 months.
    d. 24 months.

21. According to Maslow's theory of human behavior, if an individual is seeking feelings of security, stability and freedom of fear, what level of needs are they attempting to satisfy?

    a. Safety.
    b. Physiological.
    c. Social.
    d. Self-actualization.

22. A teenager who begins wetting the bed after going through a traumatic experience is likely undergoing which form of denial?

    a. Displacement.
    b. Projection.
    c. Disassociation.
    d. Regression.

23. Which of the following is an open-ended question?

    a. How did that make you feel?
    b. Are you hungry?
    c. Do you have any visual problems?
    d. Are you a nurse?

24. What is the appropriate age to initiate toilet training for the average child?

    a. 6 months.
    b. 12 months.
    c. 2 years.
    d. 4 years.

25. According to Erikson's psychosocial stages of development, which of the following people would be facing the conflict of generativity vs. stagnation?

    a. 10-year-old.
    b. 30-year-old.
    c. 45-year-old.
    d. 70-year-old.

26. A person with a substance abuse problem who argues that she is still effective in her position at work displays which forms of denial?

    a. Denial.
    b. Regression.
    c. Projection.
    d. Self-actualization.

27. Being able to explain something to someone else using simpler terms displays which of the following types of understanding?

    a. Reflection.
    b. Restatement.
    c. Clarification.
    d. Feedback.

28. When speaking to someone with an intellectual disability, which of the following is not helpful in conveying the message?

    a. Speak slowly and clearly.
    b. Limit eye contact.
    c. Use simple language.
    d. Frequently repeat yourself.

29. When taking a telephone message regarding an urgent matter, which pieces of information are most pertinent to obtain?

    a. Name, phone number, issue.
    b. Fax number, phone number, social security number.
    c. Name, insurance, issue.
    d. Issue, social security number, home address.

30. After witnessing his wife die of a heart attack, a husband blames her employer for her stressful job. The husband is in which of the following stages of grief according to Kübler-Ross?

    a. Compartmentalization.
    b. Projection.
    c. Disassociation.
    d. Anger.

31. Which of the following nonverbal cues display empathy?

    a. Relaxed posture, loud voice, limited eye contact.
    b. Rigid posture, low voice, limited eye contact.
    c. Relaxed posture, low voice, consistent eye contact.
    d. Rigid posture, loud voice, consistent eye contact.

32. A person nearby appears to be choking and having difficulty breathing. Which of the following is the initial step of care?

    a. Call 911.
    b. Ask the person if they are OK.
    c. Initiate chest compressions.
    d. Apply the Heimlich maneuver.

33. Which of the following patient's needs should be addressed first?

    a. 84-year-old man with a broken ankle.
    b. 16-year-old girl with a sore throat and fever.
    c. 65-year-old woman with chest and left arm pain.
    d. 4-year-old with a urinary tract infection.

34. What is another term for advance directive?

    a. Living will.
    b. Power of attorney.
    c. Estate representative.
    d. Legal guardian.

35. Which of the following is not part of nonverbal communication?

    a. Facial expression.
    b. Eye contact.
    c. Tone of voice.
    d. Posture.

36. In which situation would a durable power of attorney be allowed to make medical decisions for the patient?

    a. The patient is having a scheduled cesarean section.
    b. The patient has broken ribs status post mechanical fall.
    c. The patient has pneumonia.
    d. The patient is in a coma.

37. A coworker has been spotted throwing someone's medical record in the trash can in the break room. Which of the following is not an appropriate course of action?

    a. Report the action to your supervisor.
    b. Ignore the coworker's actions.
    c. Confront the coworker.
    d. Remove the records from the trash.

38. Which of the following statements is not true regarding the Americans with Disabilities Act?

    a. It helps prevent discrimination against those with disabilities.
    b. It applies only to schools and businesses.
    c. It provides reasonable accommodations to disabled persons.
    d. It prevents most employers from asking whether a person has a disability.

39. Which of the following patient's needs should be addressed last?

    a. 3-year-old with a seizure.
    b. 15-year-old with appendicitis.
    c. 26-year-old with a gunshot wound.
    d. 45-year-old with a broken wrist.

40. A doctor who accidentally amputates the wrong limb during a surgery would be guilty of which of the following?

    a. Libel.
    b. Negligence.
    c. Assault.
    d. Slander.

41. Which of the following would be overseen by the Drug Enforcement Administration (DEA)?

    a. Antihypertensive medications.
    b. Narcotics.
    c. Antiepileptic drugs.
    d. Antibiotics.

42. Which of the following is a direct question?

    a. How do you feel?
    b. How do you treat sunburn?
    c. Did you take your medication today?
    d. What type of allergic reaction did you have?

43. What is legally required prior to operating on a patient?

a. Informed consent.
b. Implied consent.
c. Expressed consent.
d. Forced consent.

44. Which of the following is not a function of the Centers for Disease Control and Prevention (CDC)?

a. Dispersing information about communicable diseases.
b. Educating about disease prevention.
c. Regulating and supervising food and medication safety.
d. Making notifications of public health emergencies.

45. Which of the following is not true regarding mental health records?

a. The practitioner is allowed to notify the person's employer.
b. The practitioner is allowed to notify law enforcement if the person is a danger to themselves or others.
c. The practitioner is allowed to share information with parents/guardians if the person is a minor.
d. The practitioner is allowed to share information with caretakers.

46. All of the following pieces of information are considered individually identifiable health information except:

a. diagnosis.
b. medical record number.
c. birth date.
d. telephone number.

47. What is the medical term for infection of the gallbladder?

a. Cholelithiasis.
b. Cholangiocarcinoma.
c. Cholecystitis.
d. Cystitis.

48. Which of the following resting heart rates signifies tachycardia?

a. 120.
b. 80.
c. 60.
d. 40.

49. A young woman who was unhappy with her physician's care decided to seek revenge by falsely accusing him of molesting her during a physical exam. What type of crime did she commit?

a. Abuse.
b. Libel.
c. Medical malpractice.
d. Assault.

50. HIPAA (Health Insurance Portability and Accountability Act) regulations apply to which of the following?

a. Physicians.
b. Secretaries.
c. Clinical documentation specialists.
d. All employees of a healthcare facility.

51. In which of the following situations should a patient not receive a medical bill?

a. A patient broke his ankle while intoxicated.
b. A patient fell down the stairs at work.
c. A patient developed a blood clot in the leg after having surgery.
d. A patient developed pneumonia while hospitalized.

52. What is the term for making a note indicating that a paper is in another file?

a. Office memo.
b. Inventory.
c. Verification.
d. Cross-reference.

53. What is the term for a complete list of items currently in the office?

a. Inventory.
b. Memo.
c. References.
d. Statistics.

54. All of the following are ways to prevent identity theft except?

a. Use the same password for all financial accounts.
b. Limit sharing personal information over the Internet.
c. Use a paper shredder for all sensitive documents.
d. Monitor credit reports on a regular basis.

55. A patient needs a referral to a specialist. Prior to referring the patient, which piece of information should be reviewed?

a. Advance directive.
b. Address.
c. Insurance.
d. Living will.

56. What is the term for when a patient requests that their health benefit payments be made directly to a designated person or facility?

a. Payment plan.
b. Advance directive.
c. Assignment of benefits.
d. Payroll.

57. Which of the following things should an office appointment calendar include?

a. Date, social security number, length of appointment.
b. Name, date, length of appointment.
c. Date, insurance provider, length of appointment.
d. Name, insurance provider, social security number.

58. What is the term for a statement sent by a health insurance company to their clients explaining what medical services were paid for on their behalf?

a. Explanation of benefits.
b. Copay.
c. Determination of benefits.
d. Deductible.

59. What is the term for the amount of money an insured client has to pay before the insurance company will pay for a claim?

a. Explanation of benefits.
b. Copay.
c. Determination of benefits.
d. Deductible.

60. What is the term for the amount of money a client must pay every time a medical service is rendered?

a. Explanation of benefits.
b. Copay.
c. Determination of benefits.
d. Deductible.

61. A patient comes to the office angrily complaining that the office did not notify her about her lab results. Which of the following is an appropriate course of action?

a. Ask the patient to leave the office.
b. Go over her lab report and explain each lab result.
c. Make a note of the complaint and call the physician.
d. Call the police to remove the patient.

62. Which of the following is the most important to ask a patient prior to a blood draw?

a. What type of insurance do you have?
b. Did you eat or drink anything today?
c. Do you write with your right hand or your left?
d. Which blood type are you?

63. When answering an office phone call, which of the following pieces of information should be given?

a. Your name, the name of the office, and the name of the physician.
b. The name of the office, the physician's name, and date.
c. Your name, the date, and the name of the physician.
d. The physician's name, the physician's phone number, and the date.

64. What is the term for assigning various tasks to those less senior?

    a. Maintenance control.
    b. Delegation.
    c. Authorization.
    d. Emancipation.

65. Which of the following is not a reason to terminate a patient-physician relationship?

    a. The patient is noncompliant with medications.
    b. The patient hasn't paid a medical bill in more than 6 months.
    c. The patient has a significant cognitive disability.
    d. The patient verbally abuses the physician and staff.

66. Which of the following is the most appropriate-sized needle to use for a routine venipuncture?

    a. 14-gauge needle.
    b. 16-gauge needle.
    c. 18-gauge needle.
    d. 20-gauge needle.

67. What is the term for assessing and treating patients by the severity of their illnesses?

    a. Advanced directive.
    b. Delegation.
    c. Staging.
    d. Triage.

68. Which of the following types of insurance plans require referrals from a primary care physician and will typically not provide coverage for providers out of network?

    a. HMO.
    b. CDS.
    c. PPO.
    d. DEA.

69. Which of the following terms refer to money owed to the physician by a patient?

    a. Accounts receivable.
    b. Payment summary.
    c. Accounts payable.
    d. Itemized bill.

70. Which of the following do not contribute to work-related injuries?

    a. Tile floors.
    b. Stepladders.
    c. Filing cabinets.
    d. Adjustable equipment.

71. A medical assistant accidentally sticks her finger with a needle after drawing blood. What is the next most appropriate step?

    a. Take an antibiotic.
    b. Continue working.
    c. Fill out an incident report.
    d. Send the needle to the lab.

72. Once a doctor decides to terminate a patient relationship, which of the following is not required?

    a. A letter from the physician to the patient.
    b. A letter from the American Medical Association to the patient.
    c. Providing the patient with their medical records.
    d. Reasonable time period to allow the patient to find another physician.

73. Which of the following would not be considered a valid petty cash purchase?

    a. Syringes.
    b. Nail polish.
    c. Computer mouse.
    d. Printer paper.

74. Which of the following is used as a part of United States Medicare reimbursement formula for physician services?

    a. Effective measure unit (EMU).
    b. Work reimbursement measure (WRM).
    c. Work value measure (WVM).
    d. Relative value unit (RVU).

75. Which of the following most accurately describes an exclusive provider organization?

    a. Wide range of doctors and hospitals to choose from.
    b. No referrals needed to see a specialist.
    c. Limited coverage for out of network services.
    d. All healthcare services go through a primary care physician.

76. Which of the following is the most appropriate step to be taken if a patient has not paid his bill in 90 days?

    a. Show up at patient's house demanding payment.
    b. Send threatening letter to the patient.
    c. Send bill to collection agency.
    d. Call patient and reprimand them.

77. Which of the following is the most appropriate definition of Medicaid?

    a. Healthcare program for college students.
    b. Healthcare program for elderly patients or those with disabilities.
    c. Healthcare program for those who are unemployed.
    d. Healthcare program for those with limited financial means.

78. What is the purpose of relative value unit (RVU)?

a. Used to help determine productivity.
b. Measures the number of certain diagnoses.
c. Calculates the possible length of hospital stay.
d. Estimates insurance rates.

79. What is the purpose of a medical waiver?

a. Permission for medical intervention.
b. Releases a person or facility from medical liability.
c. A notice that a service may not be covered by Medicare.
d. Explanation illustrating which services are covered by insurance.

80. Which of the following is the most appropriate definition of a preferred provider organization (PPO)?

a. Lower out of pocket costs but less flexibility.
b. Insurance provided by the government for low-income individuals.
c. Higher out of pocket costs but greater flexibility.
d. Insurance provided by the government for elderly individuals.

81. What is a waiver of liability?

a. A waiver that releases a person or facility from blame if an adverse event occurs.
b. A notice that a service may not be covered by Medicare.
c. Permission for medical intervention.
d. An itemized bill explaining the costs of services rendered.

82. Which of the following is the most current standard diagnostic tool to classify medical conditions into codes for the purpose of billing and reimbursement?

a. ICD-7.
b. ICD-8.
c. ICD-9.
d. ICD-10.

83. Which of the following is not a managed care organization?

a. EPO.
b. PPO.
c. HMO.
d. CEO.

84. Which of the following is not an appropriate way to manage a petty cash account?

a. Replenish once there are no more funds.
b. Set limits on expenditures.
c. Require receipts for all purchases.
d. Keep petty cash in a limited-access safe.

85. What is the term for money owed by a company to its creditors?

a. Accounts receivable.
b. Payment summary.
c. Accounts payable.
d. Itemized bill.

86. What is the purpose of the diagnosis-related group (DRG) system?

a. Monitors productivity.
b. Helps determine reimbursement.
c. Permits a physician to upcode.
d. Helps determine insurance eligibility.

87. What is the term for the breakdown of the cost for services rendered after a visit to a clinic, lab, or hospital?

a. Summary letter.
b. Itemized statement.
c. Account summary.
d. Explanation of benefits.

88. A patient sprained their wrist and had an ACE wrap placed. The physician billed for a splint placement. What is the name of this fraudulent practice?

a. Upcoding.
b. Post adjustment.
c. Bundling.
d. Accounts receivable.

89. Which of the following situations would likely result in a bundled payment?

a. Having labs drawn.
b. Getting a Pap smear.
c. Seeing a primary care physician for a follow-up visit.
d. Undergoing a cholecystectomy.

90. Which of the following is not a safety precaution when drawing blood?

a. Capping a needle when finished with the procedure.
b. Disposing of needles in a puncture-resistant biohazard container.
c. Cleaning the syringe for future use.
d. Wearing sterile gloves throughout the procedure.

91. Which of the following best describes competence?

a. Having in-depth knowledge of a particular subject.
b. Performing a task efficiently.
c. Being trustworthy.
d. Applying practical thinking to everyday situations.

92. Which of the following is not a HIPAA violation?

a. Having computer screens face into the main lobby.
b. Disclosing a patient's medical information without consent.
c. Discussing a patient's diagnosis in the waiting room.
d. Sending a patient's records to their primary care doctor's office.

93. What is the healthcare program used by the United States military?

a. PPO.
b. HMO.
c. Tricare.
d. Medicaid.

94. What is an example of a conflict of interest?

a. Accepting baseball tickets from a drug representative.
b. Making a donation to a hospital.
c. Discussing a new drug with a pharmaceutical representative.
d. Allowing medical students to rotate through the office.

95. Which of the following Healthcare Common Procedure Coding System (HCPCS) levels includes ambulance, durable medical equipment, prosthetics, orthotics and supplies when used in a physician's office?

a. I.
b. II.
c. III.
d. IV.

96. When is it appropriate to discuss a patient's case on social media?

a. If their name is not disclosed.
b. If their picture is not disclosed.
c. If their diagnosis is not disclosed.
d. It is never appropriate to discuss a patient on social media.

97. A doctor changes the medical procedure a patient received in order to obtain a higher reimbursement from the health insurance company. What is this practice called?

a. Bundling.
b. Post-adjustment.
c. Upcoding.
d. Modification.

98. What is the name for a network security system that monitors and controls the incoming and outgoing network traffic to prevent unauthorized users from accessing information?

a. Firewall.
b. Database reports.
c. Tickler file.
d. Modifiers.

99. Which of the following is not a conflict of interest?

a. Volunteering at a local homeless shelter.
b. A physician who is a board member at a pharmaceutical company.
c. Referring patients to another doctor in exchange for a monthly stipend.
d. A physician who is a promotional speaker for a medical device company.

100. Which of the following terms refers to the posterior aspect of the body?

a. Ventral.
b. Ipsilateral.
c. Lateral.
d. Dorsal.

101. What organism needs a host in order to survive?

　　a. Parasite.
　　b. Bacteria.
　　c. Virus.
　　d. Fungi.

102. Where is the liver in relation to the bladder?

　　a. Superior.
　　b. Lateral.
　　c. Ipsilateral.
　　d. Inferior.

103. What is the best way to prevent the spread of infection?

　　a. Gloves.
　　b. Hand washing.
　　c. Face mask.
　　d. Surgical gown.

104. All of the following diseases can be transmitted in the air except:

　　a. pneumonia.
　　b. influenza.
　　c. HIV.
　　d. tuberculosis.

105. Which of the following refers to the anterior aspect of the body?

　　a. Superior.
　　b. Ventral.
　　c. Dorsal.
　　d. Lateral.

106. Where is the pelvis in relation to the sternum?

　　a. Contralateral.
　　b. Ipsilateral.
　　c. Superior.
　　d. Inferior.

107. Where are the ribs in relation to the heart?

　　a. Anterior.
　　b. Posterior.
　　c. Dorsal.
　　d. Lateral.

108. What artery is most commonly used when taking blood pressure?

　　a. Femoral.
　　b. Brachial.
　　c. Subclavian.
　　d. Jugular.

109. Which of the following refers to the same side of the body?

 a. Contralateral.
 b. Lateral.
 c. Ipsilateral.
 d. Lateral recumbent.

110. What is the name of the sounds heard during measurement of a manual blood pressure?

 a. Konohoff.
 b. Kassalhoff.
 c. Katankoff.
 d. Korotkoff.

111. What information is not included in the history of present illness section of a medical chart?

 a. Onset of symptoms.
 b. Pain scale.
 c. Associated symptoms.
 d. Physical exam.

112. What is the largest organ in the human body?

 a. Liver.
 b. Lungs.
 c. Skin.
 d. Spleen.

113. Which artery is normally palpated in the wrist to take a pulse?

 a. Popliteal.
 b. Brachial.
 c. Radial.
 d. Jugular.

114. What is the most accurate measurement of body temperature?

 a. Rectal.
 b. Axillary.
 c. Temporal.
 d. Oral.

115. What piece of equipment is used for measuring blood pressure?

 a. Holter monitor.
 b. Sphygmomanometer.
 c. Urometer.
 d. Pulse oximeter.

116. What organ system is responsible for reabsorbing nutrients and excreting waste?

 a. Cardiopulmonary.
 b. Reproductive.
 c. Urinary.
 d. Endocrine.

117. What piece of equipment measures oxygen saturation?

    a. Foley catheter.
    b. Urometer.
    c. Sphygmomanometer.
    d. Pulse oximeter.

118. Which of the following would be placed in an autoclave?

    a. Scalpel.
    b. Stethoscope.
    c. Syringe.
    d. Foley catheter.

119. What organ system is responsible for taking in oxygen and excreting carbon dioxide?

    a. Neurologic.
    b. Endocrine.
    c. Integumentary.
    d. Cardiopulmonary.

120. What does the term cruris refer to?

    a. Foot.
    b. Groin.
    c. Head.
    d. Body.

121. Which of the following drugs should never be taken while pregnant?

    a. Category A.
    b. Category C.
    c. Category F.
    d. Category X.

122. Which of the following labs may be ordered to help diagnose diabetes?

    a. LDL.
    b. HbA_{1c}.
    c. Hemoglobin.
    d. TSH.

123. Morphine is used to treat which of the following?

    a. Heartburn.
    b. Nausea.
    c. Pain.
    d. High blood pressure.

124. Which instrument is used to examine ears?

    a. Ophthalmoscope.
    b. Sphygmomanometer.
    c. Otoscope.
    d. Stethoscope.

125. A patient with low hemoglobin has which condition?

    a. Anemia.
    b. Thrombocytopenia.
    c. Leukopenia.
    d. Pancytopenia.

126. A patient with a blood sugar of 36 mg/dL has which condition?

    a. Hyperkalemia.
    b. Hyperglycemia.
    c. Hypoglycemia.
    d. Hypokalemia.

127. A patient with rapid respiratory rate has which condition?

    a. Tachycardia.
    b. Bradycardia.
    c. Tachypnea.
    d. Hypotension.

128. An adipocyte is what type of cell?

    a. Fat.
    b. Bone.
    c. Brain.
    d. Skin.

129. Which of the following is the term for abnormally large breasts in men?

    a. Mastopenia.
    b. Hypergynecosis.
    c. Gynecomastia.
    d. Mastorrhea.

130. A patient who has stopped menstruating has which condition?

    a. Menarche.
    b. Dysmenorrhea.
    c. Menorrhagia.
    d. Amenorrhea.

131. What does the prefix exo- refer to?

    a. Outside.
    b. Lateral.
    c. Inside.
    d. Medial.

132. A patient with difficulty swallowing has which condition?

    a. Aphasia.
    b. Dysphagia.
    c. Aphagia.
    d. Dysphasia.

133. An osteoblast is what type of cell?

a. Bone.
b. Nerve.
c. Skin.
d. Muscle.

134. The trachea splits into which two structures?

a. Vena cava.
b. Bronchioles.
c. Alveoli.
d. Bronchi.

135. What is the medical term for inflamed or infected appendix?

a. Appendectomy.
b. Choledocholithiasis.
c. Appendicitis.
d. Cholecystectomy.

136. Which of the following procedures does not have to be done in the operating room?

a. Breast augmentation surgery.
b. Insertion of a chest tube.
c. Removal of a gallbladder.
d. Staple repair of a head laceration.

137. What structure separates the brain into the right and left sides?

a. Corpus callosum.
b. Meniscus.
c. Septum.
d. Epiglottis.

138. What procedure can evaluate the large intestine?

a. Arthroscopy.
b. Uroscopy.
c. Colonoscopy.
d. Bronchoscopy.

139. Where can a meniscus found?

a. Heart.
b. Brain.
c. Knee.
d. Spine.

140. What is the chemical symbol for sodium?

a. H.
b. Na.
c. Mg.
d. Fe.

141. Which of the following is a specialist who would treat hypothyroidism?

a. Hematologist.
b. Endocrinologist.
c. Psychiatrist.
d. Cardiologist.

142. Which condition refers to blood coming from the ear?

a. Menorrhea.
b. Dysphonia.
c. Otorrhagia.
d. Otoplasty.

143. A patient with renal failure will likely need what procedure?

a. Nephrectomy.
b. Hemodialysis.
c. Hysterectomy.
d. Urostomy.

144. What structure separates the heart into the right and left sides?

a. Vena cava.
b. Septum.
c. Ventricle.
d. Tricuspid valve.

145. A patient with brain tumor will likely need what type of specialist?

a. Gynecologist.
b. Reconstructive surgeon.
c. Hematologist.
d. Neurosurgeon.

146. What is the name of the procedure for removal of a breast?

a. Hysterectomy.
b. Polypectomy.
c. Cholecystectomy.
d. Mastectomy.

147. What is the chemical symbol for potassium?

a. K.
b. Cl.
c. P.
d. Ca.

148. Which of the following is not a common sign of a stroke?

a. Dysphagia.
b. Facial asymmetry.
c. Ataxia.
d. Rhinorrhea.

149. What is the medical term for heart attack?

a. Endocarditis.
b. Pericardial effusion.
c. Myocardial infarction.
d. Myocarditis.

150. What structure covers the trachea when a person swallows a bolus of food?

a. Hyoid.
b. Epiglottis.
c. Cruciate ligament.
d. Meniscus.

151. Which of the following is not a common finding in someone with liver failure?

a. Jaundice.
b. Confusion.
c. Abdominal distention.
d. Dysuria.

152. A patient with a deviated or "lazy" pupil has what condition?

a. Strabismus.
b. Entropion.
c. Ectropion.
d. Glaucoma.

153. What is the name of the procedure for the removal of a testicle?

a. Hysterectomy.
b. Salpinectomy.
c. Orchiectomy.
d. Oophorectomy.

154. What is the medical term for the condition "pink eye"?

a. Otitis media.
b. Conjunctivitis.
c. Cystitis.
d. Pharyngitis.

155. A patient with no heartbeat has which condition?

a. Tachycardia.
b. Asystole.
c. Bradycardia.
d. Atrial fibrillation.

156. In which of the following structures is cartilage not present?

a. Olecranon.
b. Metatarsal.
c. Patella.
d. Bladder.

157. Which of the following best describes miosis?

    a. Infection of the breast.
    b. Hearing loss.
    c. Constriction of the pupil.
    d. Excessive sweating.

158. Which of the following is not a sign of a myocardial infarction?

    a. Vision loss.
    b. Chest tightness.
    c. Shortness of breath.
    d. Jaw pain.

159. Which of the following best describes an abscess?

    a. Upper respiratory infection.
    b. Rash.
    c. Migraine.
    d. Collection of pus.

160. Which of the following is an aggressive malignant skin cancer?

    a. Melanoma.
    b. Lymphoma.
    c. Basal cell carcinoma.
    d. Glioma.

161. A patient with broken patella will likely need what type of specialist?

    a. Cardiologist.
    b. Orthopedist.
    c. Rheumatologist.
    d. Audiologist.

162. A patient with arthritis due to excessive uric acid has which condition?

    a. Glaucoma.
    b. Gout.
    c. Angina.
    d. Diverticulitis.

163. What is the name of the procedure for the removal of the foreskin on the penis?

    a. Orchiectomy.
    b. Mastectomy.
    c. Circumcision.
    d. Orchiopexy.

164. Which of the following structures is not found as a pair?

    a. Thyroid.
    b. Lung.
    c. Adrenal.
    d. Kidney.

165. Which of the following best describes a meniscus?

   a. An accessory organ attached to the intestine.
   b. A piece of cartilage between the femur and the tibia.
   c. An outpouching of the colon.
   d. A defect in the abdominal wall.

166. Which of the following organs is primarily responsible for the development of diabetes?

   a. Liver.
   b. Pancreas.
   c. Kidney.
   d. Bladder.

167. A patient with diverticulosis will likely need what type of specialist?

   a. Urologist.
   b. Gastroenterologist.
   c. Oncologist.
   d. Endocrinologist.

168. What is the medical term for presence of a kidney stone?

   a. Sialolithiasis.
   b. Cholelithiasis.
   c. Choledocholithiasis.
   d. Nephrolithiasis.

169. Which of the following best describes hepatitis?

   a. Infection of the liver.
   b. Liver malignancy.
   c. End-stage renal disease.
   d. Pancreatic malignancy.

170. What does the suffix "-pexy" mean?

   a. The presence of a malignancy.
   b. To remove something.
   c. The presence of stones.
   d. To affix something.

171. A patient with calcium deposits on the lens of the eye has which condition?

   a. Hematuria.
   b. Cataracts.
   c. Anorexia.
   d. Glaucoma.

172. Which of the following best describes cholelithiasis?

   a. Inflammation.
   b. Excessive bleeding.
   c. The presence of stones.
   d. Cessation of normal function.

173. Which of the following best describes the suffix -rrhagia?

  a. Hemorrhage.
  b. Painful.
  c. Malignancy.
  d. Infection.

174. A patient with atrial fibrillation will likely need what type of specialist?

  a. Nephrologist.
  b. Psychologist.
  c. Psychiatrist.
  d. Cardiologist.

175. What is the medical term for low urine output?

  a. Polyuria.
  b. Hematuria.
  c. Oliguria.
  d. Dysuria.

176. Which of the following best describes sickle cell anemia?

  a. Absence of red blood cells.
  b. Abnormally high number of red blood cells.
  c. Abnormally high level of iron.
  d. Abnormally shaped red blood cells.

177. A patient with a blood pressure of 165/81 mm Hg has what condition?

  a. Tachycardia.
  b. Hypotension.
  c. Hypertension.
  d. Tachypnea.

178. What does the term acetabulum refer to?

  a. Abnormal gait.
  b. Hip socket.
  c. Herniated disc.
  d. Pelvic infection.

179. A patient with excessive fatty deposits in their arteries has which condition?

  a. Atherosclerosis.
  b. Angina.
  c. Hypertension.
  d. Claudication.

180. A patient with schizophrenia will likely need what type of specialist?

  a. Psychiatrist.
  b. Gynecologist.
  c. Neonatologist.
  d. Rheumatologist.

Answers and Explanations

1. B: Food, water, sleep, and excretion are the four fundamental needs according to Maslow's hierarchy of needs. These are basic and physical needs. Next are needs of security of oneself and the safety of loved ones. The following level includes fulfillment of relationships with family members, friends, and intimacy with loved ones. Self-esteem is the second highest level, followed by the highest level of self-actualization.

2. D: Most 4-month-old babies cannot sit. Most babies at this age can coo, smile spontaneously, roll, put objects in their mouths, track with their eyes, and push themselves up on their elbows.

3. D: According to Erikson's stages of psychosocial development, children in the newborn stage to 18 months old develop trust or mistrust of their caregiver. They must have a consistent, loving caregiver present in order to form feelings of trust and a sense of safety.

4. C: Most 18-month-old children can hold a cup with assistance, walk with minimal or no assistance, follow one-step commands, show affection to familiar people, shake their head no, points to things of interest, and scribble. The other choices provided are milestones seen in older children.

5. C: Realizing one's personal potential is characteristic of the highest level in Maslow's hierarchy of needs, which is self-actualization. Self-actualization also includes the ability and desire to pursue that potential. The previous levels included in Maslow's hierarchy must usually be met prior to one's ability to reach self-actualization.

6. A: Projection is a psychological response in which a person denies his flaws or faults and instead blames them on someone else. Almost everyone does it at some point in their lives, but those with significant psychological issues may do this frequently.

7. A: Bargaining with God, a medical professional, or someone with perceived authority as an attempt to save oneself or a loved one is the third stage of grief according to Kübler-Ross. The five stages include denial, anger, bargaining, depression, and acceptance. Not all people go through all of the stages of grief. In some cases, patients return to one or more stages several times until they are able to work through it.

8. C: Speaking especially loud or yelling to a person who may not be able to hear is not appropriate. An alternative way of communicating may include hand gestures, pantomiming, writing out questions, or drawing pictures.

9. A: Weather is an external barrier to communication, as it may cause a distraction that draws the listener or speaker's attention away from the message being sent. Internal barriers are issues or problems that are occurring within the person such as stress, anger, hunger, depression, or pain. These issues can affect concentration and mental processes.

10. A: Most 12- to 18-year-olds face identity versus role confusion per Erikson's stages of psychosocial development. Through the development of peer relationships and social groups, children and adolescents must find their sense of self through hobbies, occupation, politics, and religion.

11. A: Reflection is having a deep enough understanding of a particular lesson that one is able to draw correlations to personal experiences in one's own life.

12. A: Food, water, sleep, and excretion are the four fundamental physiological needs according to Maslow's hierarchy of needs. These are the basic and physical needs that must first be fulfilled in order for the individual to be able to fulfill the subsequent needs in Maslow's hierarchy of needs.

13. B: Disassociation is a psychological defense mechanism where a person mentally separates themselves from a significantly painful experience. They may do this by creating separate personalities, by daydreaming, or developing amnesia.

14. D: Loss of interest in hobbies, avoidance of social events, withdrawal from loved ones, and pervasive feelings of anxiety and unhappiness are signs of depression. It is the fourth stage of grief according to Kübler-Ross. The five stages include denial, anger, bargaining, depression, and acceptance. Grief itself is not a stage in Kübler-Ross's stages of grief.

15. C: According to Erikson's stages of psychosocial development, most elementary-aged children face industry versus inferiority. They must master new emotional, educational, and social skills. If they fail to do so, they develop feelings of insecurity and failure.

16. C: A rigid versus a relaxed posture denotes tense feelings, anger, and aggressiveness. Sudden movements or gestures can convey hostility. Standing in close proximity can mean intimacy; however, when seen with other cues such as rigid posture and sudden movements, it conveys aggressiveness and desire for possible physical conflict.

17. B: Following five commands in a row would be seen in a 7- or 8-year-old, rather than a 5-year-old. Five-year-olds generally have good motor control and can skip, hop, and jump with little difficulty. They have a fairly large vocabulary of around 2,000 words. They can memorize basic facts such as address, names, and ages of close family members, and their telephone number.

18. A: Older toddlers to those about to enter kindergarten face initiative versus guilt. They are becoming more independent and assertive but becoming excessively so may cause feelings of guilt and anxiety.

19. C: A person who is chronically homeless is likely very hungry. This kind of internal barrier may affect effective communication. Internal barriers are issues or problems that are occurring within the person such as stress, anger, hunger, depression, or pain. These issues can affect concentration and mental processes.

20. B: While there is a wide age range when children begin to crawl, the typical range is 6 to 10 months. Babies who are 3 months are just learning to pick up their heads without assistance. If a child is not crawling by 18 months, further investigation and workup is warranted.

21. A: Maslow's need of safety includes the security of oneself and the safety of loved ones. Individuals seeking to satisfy their need of safety are seeking freedom from their fears, stability in their life and in their relationships, and protection from things that threaten themselves and those they love.

22. D: Regression is a defense mechanism where a person may go back to a period in their lives when they felt safer and did not have to face the particular traumatic event. An example of this could be a teenager who starts wetting the bed or an adult who starts throwing temper tantrums like a toddler.

23. A: An open-ended question requires an answer with some detailed explanation or depth. A closed or a direct question only requires one-word answers such as yes or no.

24. C: While there is a wide age range when children can initiate toilet training, most are generally considered appropriate for this task between 2 and 3 years of age. At this point they have enough understanding to do what is asked and likely have the capacity to hold their bowels or bladder for a short period of time.

25. C: People who are in middle adulthood around 45 to 60 years of age face generativity versus stagnation. People want to create and accomplish things before they may retire or die. They want to nurture their children to become functional adults in society. Failure to do these things may make people become withdrawn from society and from their family members.

26. A: Denial is a psychological defense mechanism in which people attempt to rationalize their flaws or problems. It is a way for people to deny or minimize the seriousness of the issue.

27. B: Restatement is a way of explaining things in a person's own words in simpler terms than the original explanation. This prevents plagiarism and illustrates that the person truly understands the idea enough to explain it to others.

28. B: Limiting eye contact is not helpful when trying to communicate to someone with a learning disability. Maintaining consistent eye contact may help engage the individual and help them understand what is being explained.

29. A: Obtaining a person's name, their contact information, such as an email address, phone number, or fax number, and a brief message summarizing the issue are the most important pieces of information when transcribing an urgent matter. Things such as social security number or home address may be of importance, but these things can be obtained later. Asking for insurance information may delay addressing the issue at hand.

30. D: The husband is displaying anger, which is the second stage of grief. He is misplacing his strong emotional feelings on another person as a way of emotional release. The five stages of grief include denial, anger, bargaining, depression, and acceptance.

31. C: A relaxed versus a rigid posture creates feelings of ease, trust, and serenity. Using a low voice in a reassuring tone helps contribute to that atmosphere. Maintaining consistent eye contact improves communication and helps build feelings of trust.

32. B: Asking the person if they are OK is the best initial step. If they are unable to speak or just shake their head, call 911. If they are choking and are unable to speak, initiate the Heimlich maneuver. If they lose consciousness, begin chest compressions.

33. C: Any person with a potentially life-threatening injury should be addressed first. Chest and left arm pain can signify a heart attack. People with suspected heart attacks, strokes, aneurysmal dissections, pulmonary embolus, or other severe emergencies need to be taken care of immediately because the mortality rates in these cases are very high. Those with injuries such as a broken ankle or medical issues such as a sore throat are important, but typically are not life-threatening.

34. A: A living will is an advance directive. It usually names a power of attorney who is someone that will verbalize their wishes and can make medical decisions if the patient is unable to speak for him/herself. It also usually dictates the type of interventions the patient does or does not want. For example, a person may not want to be intubated, receive dialysis, or receive life-saving measures if they are not expected to have a full recovery.

35. C: Tone of voice is a type of verbal communication. Gestures, posture, facial expression, proximity, and eye contact are all nonverbal types of communication.

36. D: When a patient is in a coma or is otherwise unable to verbalize his/her wishes, the power of attorney becomes the advocate for the patient. This person is usually named in a person's living will or advance directive. If no living will exists, a spouse, parent, or child (depending on the circumstances and family situation) will be assigned the power of attorney. If no friends or family are present, the medical facility will designate a power of attorney for the patient through legal channels.

37. B: Ignoring someone who is doing something illegal, unethical, or immoral is not appropriate. The action should be addressed by someone. It is reasonable to confront the person yourself. It is equally reasonable to go directly to a supervisor and have them address the issue. In this case, since the medical records were not properly disposed of, they should be removed from the trash can and be placed in a proper hospital-designated trash receptacle.

38. B: The Americans with Disabilities Act (ADA) applies to everyone, including schools, all types of businesses, and employers. It helps prevent against discrimination in the workplace and allows those with disabilities to participate as active members in society.

39. D: While a broken wrist may be a big inconvenience and should be addressed in a timely manner, urgent or life-threatening cases should always be evaluated first. People with seizures, gunshot wounds, acute appendicitis, or other severe emergencies need to be taken care of immediately because the mortality and complication rates in these cases can be high.

40. B: Negligence is a complication or death that has occurred because of carelessness. Failure to properly review the chart and mark the limb scheduled for amputation is a negligent act. The doctor did not mean to cause harm, but failed to act with prudence.

41. B: The DEA is a federal law enforcement agency that is in charge of dealing with controlled pharmaceuticals and illegal drugs. For example, a medical practitioner who sells narcotic pain medications to patients or the general public would be investigated by the DEA.

42. C: Questions that can be answered with a yes, no, or a one-word reply are considered direct questions. Questions that require a more detailed response are open-ended questions.

43. A: Informed consent must be obtained from a person or their power of attorney prior to a procedure. This includes explaining the procedure itself, the need for the procedure, and any risks associated with the procedure. Consent is usually signed with one or more witnesses (usually nursing staff) prior to the procedure taking place.

44. C: The regulation and supervision of food and medication safety is controlled by the Food and Drug Administration (FDA). The Centers for Disease Control and Prevention (CDC) is in charge of the dissemination of information about communicable diseases, vaccine advocacy, and education of public awareness.

45. A: Unless the person in question poses a risk to their employer or threatens violence in their workplace, the medical practitioner is not allowed to notify their place of employment. If a person does pose a risk to themselves or others, the medical professional is obligated to contact the person(s) in potential danger and the local authorities.

46. A: A diagnosis does not identify a particular individual. Millions of people may have the same diagnosis. Pieces of information such as name, date of birth, social security number, address, medical record number, and telephone number may be used to identify a particular individual.

47. C: Cholecystitis is an infection of the gallbladder. The suffix -itis means inflammation and the term cholecyst means relating to the gallbladder.

48. A: Tachycardia refers to an abnormally fast heart rate. The average adult human heart rate is 60 to 100 beats per minute. The prefix tachy- means fast. A resting heart rate that exceeds 100 beats per minute is considered tachycardic.

49. B: Libel is a crime in which someone knowingly makes a false statement in the hopes of damaging someone's reputation or credibility. Libel is the written form of this crime whereas slander is spread through word of mouth.

50. D: HIPAA (Health Insurance Portability and Accountability Act) requires that all employees of a medical facility maintain patient confidentiality, no matter what role they play in the patient's care.

51. B: The patient who obtained their injury at their place of employment is eligible for workers' compensation. This form of insurance means the employer pays the medical bill.

52. D: Cross-referencing is when a note or file shows that paperwork can be found in another file. It identifies where more information can be found elsewhere.

53. A: An inventory is a complete list of supplies and the numbers of each that are currently in the office. This will help keep track of when and how many items need to be replenished.

54. A: Identity theft is becoming increasingly common as more information is publicized and stored on the Internet. To prevent against identity left, passwords should all be different and contain a combination of upper- and lower-case letters, numbers, and characters. Limit the amount and type of personal information shared on the Internet. Use a shredder for bills or sensitive documents that contain personal information. Obtain a credit report at least twice a year to monitor credit activity.

55. C: The patient's insurance carrier should be reviewed. Some patients need a referral prior to going to a specialist while others may not. Some patients will not be covered if they go out of network while others may be covered. Some specialists accept only certain insurance carriers.

56. C: Assignment of benefits is an authorization from an insured to allow any payment to go directly to the physician. The payment of their benefit can be given directly to the doctor or the treating facility so they can apply the benefit payment to the debt owed by the patient.

57. B: The most important pieces of information are the patient's name, date of the appointment, and length of the appointment. If it is a new consultation, that appointment will likely run longer than a routine follow-up. Social security number and insurance carrier are not needed in the appointment calendar. A patient's social security number should never be displayed on a public document.

58. A: An explanation of benefits (EOB) letter explains to insured individuals which medical services and treatments were paid for by the insurance company. It identifies the amount charged by the provider(s), the amount paid for by the insurance company, and the amount for which the client is responsible.

59. D: A deductible is a set amount of money set by the health care insurance company that has to be paid by the client before the company pays for a claim. The amount will differ by company and by individual depending on the type of policy that they own.

60. B: A copay is an amount of money set by the health care insurance company that needs to be paid by the client every time a medical service is rendered. For example, a patient may need to pay $20 every time she visits her primary care physician.

61. C: The most appropriate course of action is to try to keep the patient calm, show empathy, and document the complaint. Let the patient know that the physician will be notified and will review the lab results with the patient at the first available opportunity. Having the patient removed from the office if they are not being violent or making threats against the staff is not appropriate. The medical assistant should not explain the results of the labs; that responsibility should fall on the physician.

62. B: Asking if patients ate or drank anything is important because it indicates whether or not they may faint during or following the procedure. If they did not have anything to eat or drink, have them recline or lie down. Ask them drink juice after the blood is drawn but before they leave the office to prevent an episode of syncope later.

63. A: When answering the office phone, the standard greeting should include your name, the name of the office, and the physician's name. The patient likely knows the date and does not need the phone number because they are the one calling the office.

64. B: Delegating responsibilities is when a senior authority assigns tasks to those working for her/him. This allows work to be completed in a timelier manner and maximizes productivity.

65. C: A physician may not terminate a patient relationship due to a physical or cognitive disability. The Americans with Disabilities Act (ADA) applies to all types of businesses, including schools, medical facilities, clinics, and employers. It helps prevent against discrimination in the workplace and in society.

66. D: The lower the needle gauge, the larger the bore of the needle. Large bore IVs should be used for trauma patients or in emergent situations only. Small bore needles should be used for routine venipunctures. A 20- to 25-gauge needle should be used in routine procedures.

67. D: Triaging patients is when a medical provider treats the most critical cases first. A life-threatening injury such as a gunshot wound would take priority over a broken ankle. Although a broken ankle is painful and inconvenient, it does not present imminent danger to the patient.

68. A: HMOs require coordinating all health care through a primary care physician (PCP). If a specialist is needed, the patient would first have to visit his PCP in order to obtain a referral. This type of insurance coverage usually is less expensive.

69. A: Accounts receivable is money owed to a company by its debtors. In this case it is the money owed to the physician by the patient.

70. D: Tile flooring is a safety hazard because of its slick surface. It increases the risk of falls and injuries. Stepladders prevent the staff from using a rolling chair or a piece of unsafe equipment in order to reach something. Filing cabinets allow items to be stored safely as opposed to leaving them in boxes on the floor. Adjustable equipment helps prevent against ergonomic injuries.

71. C: An incident report is a detailed account of an injury that occurred in a healthcare setting. An antibiotic may or may not be used due to the extent of the injury. The medical assistant should stop working immediately and fill out an incident report and seek medical attention. Sending the needle to the lab would not be helpful. Certain infectious diseases such as AIDS do not survive in the air. The medical assistant should have her blood drawn to screen for infectious diseases and to determine whether she needs prophylactic therapy.

72. B: A letter from the American Medical Association is not required for the termination of a patient-physician relationship. A letter from the physician with an effective date of termination is required. The date should allow reasonable time for the patient to find another provider. The provider should also give the patient a copy of their medical records so the new provider can be familiar with their medical history.

73. B: Nail polish is not a valid office expense. Petty cash is meant for office-related purchases that may be due to a last-minute need. For example, if there is no more printer paper, a staff member may be asked to go out and buy more.

74. D: Relative value units (RVUs) are part of the system Medicare uses to decide how much it will reimburse physicians for services rendered. Since RVUs help measure productivity, they can also be used as a tool to help multi-physician practices determine how much to pay their physicians.

75. B: Exclusive provider organizations (EPOs) combine affordability with flexibility. No primary care physician referrals are needed to see specialists. However, there is a limited network to choose from and there is usually no coverage for out of network services.

76. C: Send the overdue payment to a collection agency. Calling the patient with threats or showing up at their house can be considered harassment.

77. D: Medicaid is a social healthcare program for those with limited financial means or who have certain disabilities. It is used for those who are permanent legal residents or US citizens to obtain health care and services.

78. A: Relative value units (RVUs) are part of the system Medicare uses to decide how much it will reimburse physicians for services rendered. Since RVUs help measure productivity, they can also be used as a tool to help multi-physician practices determine how much to pay their physicians.

79. B: A medical waiver is signed by a person or their power of attorney, releasing a person or facility from medical liability. For example, a pediatrician may make a parent sign a medical waiver prior to administering vaccinations. Another example would be a sky diving instructor having a patient with a heart condition sign a waiver prior to jumping out of the plane.

80. C: Preferred provider organizations (PPOs) have larger out of pocket costs but have greater flexibility. A primary care physician is not needed in order to see a specialist. A person may visit an out of network provider or facility and be covered, although the coverage is less than if they stayed in network.

81. B: An Advance Beneficiary Notice (ABN), also known as a waiver of liability, is a notice you should receive when a provider offers you a service they believe Medicare will not cover.

82. D: International Classification of Diseases (ICD-10) codes are the most current diagnostic tool used to classify medical conditions for the purpose of billing a reimbursement. ICD-10 codes replaced ICD-9 codes in the fall of 2015.

83. D: The three major types of managed care organizations are preferred provider organizations (PPO), exclusive provider organization (EPO), and health maintenance organization (HMO). A CEO is a chief executive officer or the head of an organization.

84. A: Petty cash funds should be replenished once the money is low, but not completely gone. Petty cash is meant for office-related purchases that may be due to a last-minute need. For example, if there is no more printer paper, a staff member may be asked to go out and buy more.

85. C: Accounts payable is the term for money owed by a company to its creditors. For example, a medical office may owe money to the utility company for providing electricity to the office.

86. B: The diagnosis-related group divides diagnoses into almost two dozen body systems, which have several hundred subdivisions. These help sort medical conditions to determine Medicare reimbursement.

87. B: An itemized bill is a breakdown of services that were provided to the patient and the cost for each service rendered. This helps the patient understand their bill better and minimizes confusion.

88. A: When a provider upcodes, they assign a code for a more expensive service or procedure than what was performed. This is a fraudulent practice that will result in legal ramifications as well as inappropriate future medical management because the patient's past medical history has been altered.

89. D: A bundled payment covers services delivered by two or more providers during a single episode of care or over a single period of time. A person undergoing a cholecystectomy will be charged by the hospital for the hospital stay, by the surgeon, and by the anesthesiologist. Instead of receiving multiple bills, all charges are bundled into a single payment.

90. C: Syringes should not be reused, especially if a patient is having a blood draw. Syringes, needles, bloody gauzes, and other contaminated equipment should be disposed of properly to prevent injury and prevent the spread of infectious diseases.

91. B: Competence is the ability to perform a task effectively and efficiently. A person who is competent meets the minimum standards of expectations for their job.

92. D: Sending a patient's medical records to their primary care doctor's office is not a HIPAA violation. It is necessary to maintain a continuity of care after a patient has seen a specialist for a new problem or has been recently been hospitalized.

93. C: Tricare is the healthcare program used by the United States military. It provides healthcare coverage for active and retired military personnel and their dependents.

94. A: A conflict of interest is when a person's involvement with another person or another organization may corrupt the care of their patients. For example, accepting money or gifts from pharmaceutical or medical equipment representatives is a conflict of interest. The representative may use their gifts to influence a physician's decision to prescribe a certain medication or use a certain product.

95. B: HCPCS codes are used to describe medical and diagnostic procedures and bill Medicare. There are three levels of codes. Level II includes ambulance, durable medical equipment, prosthetics, orthotics, and supplies when used in a physician's office.

96. D: Discussing a patient or any aspect of their case on social media is a violation of HIPAA. HIPAA requires that all employees of a medical facility maintain patient confidentiality.

97. C: When a provider upcodes, they assign a code for a more expensive service or procedure than was performed. This is a fraudulent practice that will result in legal ramifications as well as inappropriate future medical management because a patient's past medical history has been altered.

98. A: A firewall is a computer security system that helps protects patients' sensitive documents and information. This helps physicians and their staff members comply with HIPAA.

99. A: A conflict of interest is when a person's involvement with another person or another organization may corrupt the care of their patients. A physician who received a stipend from another physician for referrals, being a promotional speaker for a certain product, or having a financial investment in a particular drug may alter a physician's care in order to obtain financial gain.

100. D: The dorsum of an object refers to the posterior or back part. Ventral or anterior means the front of something. Ipsilateral means the same side. Lateral is next to or on the side of something.

101. A: A parasite is an organism that lives in or on a host and siphons nutrients as well as other benefits in order to survive. An example would the tapeworm, which is transmitted through the fecal-oral route. It lives in the gut and absorbs food and nutrients, leaving the host hungry and malnourished.

102. A: The liver is in the right upper quadrant of the abdomen. The bladder is in the abdominopelvic region. The liver is above or superior to the bladder. The bladder is below or inferior to the liver. Ipsilateral means the same side. Lateral is next to or on the side of something.

103. B: Although all of the choices are excellent measures to help prevent the spread of infection, hand washing is the number one way to help prevent the spread of disease. Medical practitioners should be using soap and water or alcohol sanitizer throughout the day.

104. C: HIV/AIDS is a disease that is not transmitted in the air. The virus dies in the air quickly. It is transmitted through bodily fluids. It may be passed to others via contaminated needles, blood, and sexual contact with an infected partner.

105. B: The front (anterior) portion of the body is referred to as the ventral aspect. The superior aspect is the top portion. The dorsal side may be referred to as posterior. Lateral is next to or on the side of something.

106. D: The pelvis is in the pelvic cavity, which is beneath or inferior to the sternum. The sternum is also known as the breast bone, which is located in the thoracic cavity. The sternum is above or superior to the pelvis. Contralateral means opposite side. Ipsilateral means the same side.

107. A: The ribs are anterior or in front of the heart. Conversely the heart is posterior or dorsal to the ribs. Lateral refers to something being next to or adjacent to something else. For example, the ulna is lateral to the radius.

108. B: The brachial artery can be palpated on the ventral surface of the arm anterior to the elbow. The blood pressure cuff or sphygmomanometer and a stethoscope can be used to help measure blood pressure by auscultating Korotkoff sounds. Systolic pressure is registered as the pressure at which the sounds are first heard, and diastolic as the pressure at which they disappear.

109. C: Ipsilateral refers to being on the same side or plane. For example, the right arm is ipsilateral to the right leg. Contralateral refers to being on the same side. Lateral means adjacent to something. Lateral recumbent is a body position where a person lies on their side with their contralateral leg flexed.

110. D: The blood pressure cuff or sphygmomanometer and a stethoscope can be used to help measure blood pressure by auscultating Korotkoff sounds. Systolic pressure is registered as the pressure at which the sounds are first heard, and diastolic as the pressure at which they disappear.

111. D: The history of present illness (HPI) includes subjective information that the patient gives to the medical practitioner such as chief complaint, associated symptoms, pain quality, and scale. The HPI also includes past medical history, past surgical history, social history, family history, allergies, and medications. The physical exam contains objective findings seen by the medical professional.

112. C: The skin is considered an organ and it is the largest organ in the human body. The skin is only a few millimeters thick yet is by far the largest organ in the body. It helps protect the body organs from trauma, extreme temperatures, fluid losses, and infection.

113. C: The radial and ulnar arteries are found in the wrist and are used when a practitioner is taking a pulse in a clinic. The popliteal artery is found in the leg posterior to the knee. The brachial artery is commonly palpated in the antecubital fossa, which is anterior to the elbow. The jugular artery is in the neck.

114. A: Temperatures taken from within a body cavity are much more accurate than those taken from a body surface. Oral temperatures can be fairly accurate, but in some circumstances may not be able to be taken properly. An oral temperature may not be accurate if a patient is intubated or is a young child. In those cases, a rectal temperature is best.

115. B: The blood pressure cuff or sphygmomanometer and a stethoscope can be used to help measure blood pressure by auscultating Korotkoff sounds. Systolic pressure is registered as the pressure at which the sounds are first heard, and diastolic as the pressure at which they disappear.

116. C: The urinary system helps excrete waste products and reabsorbs nutrients and water if a person is dehydrated. The kidneys help filter toxins from the body and eliminate them via urine.

117. D: A pulse oximeter (also known as a "pulse ox") can be placed on a finger, ear, or toe, and helps measure oxygen saturation. It is usually seen on telemetry floors and in the intensive care unit.

118. A: Autoclaves sterilize equipment that is meant to be reused, but has been in contact with bodily fluids. They use high-temperature steam or heat to kill off organisms. Autoclaves are typically used for operating room equipment such as scalpels. Syringes, needles, and Foley catheters are meant for single person use. Stethoscopes should be cleaned with alcohol wipes periodically. They will be destroyed in an autoclave.

119. D: The cardiopulmonary system takes in oxygen during inspiration and distributes it to the body and tissues. It excretes carbon dioxide, which is released from the body during expiration.

120. B: Cruris refers to groin. For example, tinea cruris means a fungal rash of the groin. Pedis refers to foot, capitus refers to head, and corporis refers to the body.

121. D: Category X drugs are expected to cause deformities in a fetus and should never be used in pregnancy. The Food and Drug Administration established five categories to indicate the potential of a drug to cause birth defects in pregnant women. Category A drugs have been shown in studies to not cause fetal deformities. In Category B drugs, animal reproduction studies have failed to demonstrate a risk to the fetus. Category C drugs have demonstrated that they may cause harm to the fetus in animal reproduction studies. Many antiepileptic drugs fall into this category. However, because seizures also cause harm to the fetus and mother, the risks and benefits must be carefully considered. Category D drugs have demonstrated that they may cause harm to the fetus in human reproduction studies.

122. B: Glycated hemoglobin (HbA$_{1c}$) measures the average blood glucose level over the previous 3 months. It helps diagnose diabetes. Low-density lipoprotein is a measure of cholesterol in the body. Hemoglobin helps measure the level of blood in the body. Thyroid-stimulating hormone helps measure thyroid abnormalities.

123. C: Morphine is a narcotic medicine used to treat moderate to severe pain. It should be used with caution because it can cause central nervous system depression if a patient is given too much.

124. C: An otoscope is used to examine someone's ears. An ophthalmoscope is used to examine eyes. The blood pressure cuff or sphygmomanometer and a stethoscope can be used to help measure blood pressure.

125. A: Anemia means the hemoglobin level is low. There are multiple causes, including acute blood loss, iron deficiency, and diseases such as sickle cell anemia. The goal of treatment is to correct the underlying cause.

126. C: Hypoglycemia means blood glucose is low. A normal sugar range is 70 to 120 mg/dL. Hyperkalemia is an elevated potassium level. Hyperglycemia is an elevated blood glucose level. Hypokalemia is an abnormally low potassium level.

127. C: Tachypnea is an elevated respiratory rate. A normal respiratory rate is 12 to 20 breaths per minute. Tachycardia is an elevated heart rate. Bradypnea is a decreased respiratory rate. Hypotension is low blood pressure.

128. A: Adipocytes make up adipose or fat tissue. Adipo means fat and -cyte means cell. An osteocyte is a bone cell. Glial cells and neurons can be found in the nervous system.

129. C: Gynecomastia is the presence of abnormally large breast tissue in men. This may due to obesity or hormonal imbalances. The goal of treatment is to correct the underlying cause.

130. D: Amenorrhea is the absence of a menstrual period. It may be due to pregnancy, infertility issues, hormonal imbalance, or the onset of menopause. Menarche is a woman's first menses. Dysmenorrhea refers to a painful period. Menorrhagia refers to a period with heavy flow.

131. A: The prefix exo- refers to the outside or exterior of something. An exoskeleton is an exterior skeleton that protects the body's inner structures; crabs and lobsters are examples. Exocrine glands secrete hormones through ducts that open into the epithelium rather than directly into the bloodstream.

132. B: A patient with dysphagia has difficulty swallowing. The prefix dys- means abnormal irregular, or difficult. The prefix a- means without or absent. The suffix -phagia refers to the act of swallowing. The suffix -phasia refers to speech.

133. A: An osteoblast refers to a bone cell. It is a specialized type of bone cell that makes bone. It does so by producing a matrix that then becomes mineralized. Osteoclasts are other specialized types of bone cells that break down the bony matrix.

134. D: The trachea splits into two structures called the right bronchus and left bronchus. The bronchi branch out further into bronchioles that separate into alveoli, which are tiny air sacs. The vena cava is a large vein that carries oxygen to the heart.

135. C: Appendicitis is an inflamed or infected appendix. The word append- refers to the appendix. The suffix -otomy means to surgically remove. The term choledocho- refers to the common bile duct. Chole- refers to the gallbladder. The suffix -lithiasis means the abnormal presence of stones.

136. D: Staple or suture repair of the head can be done as a bedside procedure. The other three choices should be done in an operating room in a controlled environment because they involve operating within a body cavity. Anesthesia needs to be administered, vital signs need to be monitored, and a sterile field needs to be in place.

137. A: The corpus callosum is a thick band of nerve fibers that connects the right cerebral hemisphere to the left. It is used to transmit messages between the right and left halves of the brain. A meniscus is a crescent-shaped cartilage found between the femur and tibia that acts as a shock absorber. The septum separates the right and left sides of the heart. The epiglottis is a piece of cartilage that closes off the trachea while swallowing or the esophagus when breathing.

138. C: A colonoscopy is a procedure done under general anesthesia that allows physicians to evaluate the rectum and large intestine for diseases or malignancy. An arthroscopy evaluates the joint space. Uroscopy evaluates the bladder. A bronchoscopy evaluates the large airways.

139. C: A meniscus is a crescent-shaped cartilage found between the femur and tibia that acts as a shock absorber. There is a lateral meniscus and a medial meniscus. If one or both are damaged, a patient may experience chronic knee pain. A meniscal tear can be diagnosed with an arthroscopy.

140. B: The chemical symbol for sodium is Na. The symbol for hydrogen is H. The symbol for magnesium is Mg. The chemical symbol for iron is Fe.

141. B: An endocrinologist is a specialist who treats hormonal disorders of the endocrine system. The thyroid is a major endocrine gland. A hematologist treats disorders of the blood. A psychiatrist treats those who have mental or emotional disorders. A cardiologist specializes in issues pertaining to the heart.

142. C: Otorrhagia refers to a hemorrhage from the ear. Oto- refers to the ear. The suffix -rrhagia refers to heavy flow. The prefix dys- means abnormal irregular or difficult. Dysphonia means a problem with one's voice; this can occur in patients with laryngitis. The prefix a- means without or absent. Amenorrhea is an absence or lack of menstrual flow. The suffix -plasty means surgical repair. Otoplasty is a surgical repair of the ear.

143. B: Hemodialysis would be needed in those with end-stage renal failure. The kidneys have many important functions. One of these functions is to filter toxins from the blood. When the kidneys are not working properly, the toxins can accumulate within the body and cause infection and potentially death. In order to prevent these complications, a patient is hooked up to an external machine that filters out the toxins. Essentially it acts like an external kidney. This process is called hemodialysis.

144. B: The septum is a dividing wall between the right and left sides of the heart. This helps keep the oxygenated blood on the left side away from the deoxygenated blood on the right side.

145. D: A neurosurgeon is a surgical specialist who is trained in the disorders of the brain and spine. A gynecologist is a physician who specializes in the female reproductive tract. A reconstructive surgeon or a plastic surgeon specializes in augmentation of the body or repair. A hematologist specializes in disorders of the blood.

146. D: A mastectomy is a surgical removal of the breast, usually due to malignancy. A hysterectomy involves the removal of the uterus. A polypectomy is the removal of a polyp. A polyp is a pedunculated piece of tissue that can grow within an organ. It is usually seen in the colon, but can also be found in other areas such as the uterus. Polyps can be benign or malignant. A cholecystectomy is the surgical removal of the gallbladder.

147. A: The chemical symbol for potassium is K. Cl signifies chloride. The chemical symbol P means phosphorus. Ca signifies calcium.

148. D: Rhinorrhea means watery nasal discharge or runny nose. The symptoms can be seen in allergic reactions, stress, and upper respiratory infections, but is not a sign of a stroke. Signs of stroke may include dysarthria, ataxia, facial droop, ptosis, and aphasia.

149. C: The medical term for a heart attack is a myocardial infarction. A heart attack occurs when the cardiac cells in a portion of the heart die due to prolonged insufficient blood and oxygen flow. Signs and symptoms may include chest pain, shortness of breath, palpitations, diaphoresis, nausea, vomiting, dizziness, and feeling of impending doom.

150. B: The epiglottis is a piece of cartilage that protects both the trachea and the esophagus. It covers the trachea when swallowing food to help prevent aspiration. It covers the esophagus when breathing to ensure the oxygen is being dispersed to the lungs and tissues and the carbon dioxide is being released to the environment.

151. D: Dysuria is painful urination. It is usually seen in those with urinary tract infections (UTIs). Although UTIs can occur in someone with liver failure, it is not a symptom of liver failure itself. Jaundice is a yellowing of the skin and mucosa. It is due to excessive bilirubin, a yellow pigment in the blood. It is normally broken down by the liver. The liver helps filter toxins, and a patient may become confused when the liver is not functioning (encephalopathy). Liver abnormalities also alter albumin and salt levels, causing fluid retention and abdominal distention called ascites.

152. A: Strabismus is a deviated pupil (can be medial or lateral) also known as lazy eye. Entropion is the turning inward of the eyelid. Conversely ectropion is the outward turning of the eyelid. Glaucoma is a condition in which the intraocular pressure is increased, causing pain, redness, and vision loss.

153. C: An orchiectomy is the removal of a testicle. This procedure may be due to malignancy or severe trauma. Oophorectomy is the removal of the ovaries. Hysterectomy is the removal of the uterus. Salpingectomy is the removal of one or both Fallopian tubes.

154. B: The conjunctiva is the white part of the eye. The suffix -itis refers to inflammation or infection. Cystitis is the infection of the bladder. A sore throat due to bacteria or a virus is called pharyngitis. Otitis media is an infection of the middle ear.

155. B: Asystole is a condition in which no heartbeat is present. The prefix a- means without and the word systole means the contraction phase during a cardiac cycle. Bradycardia is an abnormally slow heart rate. A normal heart rate is 60 to 100 beats per minute. Atrial fibrillation is an irregular heartbeat. Tachycardia is an abnormally fast heart rate.

156. D: Cartilage is a thin, soft connective tissue commonly found between bones within the joint. It is seen in the olecranon (elbow), metatarsal (foot), and patella (knee). Cartilage is not found in the bladder.

157. C: Miosis is the constriction or narrowing of the pupil. The pupil is the black part of the eye that helps regulate light. In a very well-lit area, the pupil will constrict. In dimly lit areas, it will dilate. Certain drugs such as narcotics may also cause miosis.

158. A: Vision loss is not a sign of a heart attack (myocardial infarction). A heart attack occurs when the cardiac cells in a portion of the heart die due to prolonged insufficient blood and oxygen flow. Signs and symptoms may include chest pain, shortness of breath, jaw pain, palpitations, diaphoresis, nausea, vomiting, dizziness, and feeling of impending doom.

159. D: An abscess is a collection of pus underneath the skin or in a body or brain cavity caused by one or more bacteria. Simples abscesses found in the superficial layers of the skin may be treated with antibiotics by mouth and incision and drainage. Complex abscesses found in sensitive areas (such as the rectum) or in a body cavity or the brain require intravenous antibiotics and surgical debridement.

160. A: Melanoma is an aggressive form of skin cancer. A glioma is a malignancy found in the glial cells in the central nervous system. Basal cell carcinoma is the most common type of skin cancer. It is highly treatable with an excellent prognosis because it is very slow growing. Lymphomas are a malignancy of the lymphatic system.

161. B: A broken patella (kneecap) would have to be evaluated by an orthopedist. An orthopedist is a physician who specializes in the musculoskeletal system. A rheumatologist is a physician who specializes in musculoskeletal autoimmune disorders such as rheumatoid arthritis. An audiologist deals with hearing dysfunction. A cardiologist focuses on structural heart abnormalities and cardiac arrhythmias.

162. B: Gout is a condition characterized by uric acid deposits in the joints causing inflammation, pain, and swelling. Angina is chest pain that may occur at rest or be precipitated by activity. Diverticulosis is the presence of small outpouchings in the colon usually caused by a low-fiber diet. Glaucoma is caused by increased intraocular pressure leading to pain, erythema, and blindness.

163. C: Circumcision involves removing the foreskin of the penis (usually done in male infants) for medical and/or religious reasons. Orchiopexy involves affixing one or both testicles in a certain position, or correcting testicular torsion. A male child with an undescended testicle after 1 year of age would undergo an orchiopexy. An orchiectomy is the removal of a testicle due to malignancy or severe trauma. A mastectomy is the removal of a breast usually due to malignancy.

164. A: There are two lobes to the thyroid gland, but there is only one thyroid. Lungs, adrenal glands, and kidneys are present in pairs.

165. B: A meniscus is a crescent-shaped cartilage found between the femur and tibia that acts as a shock absorber. There is a lateral meniscus and a medial meniscus. If one or both are damaged, a patient may experience chronic knee pain.

166. B: The pancreas is involved in the development of diabetes. The pancreas contains the islets of Langerhans. The beta cells on the islets of Langerhans produce insulin. In type 1 diabetes, the immune system attacks the islets of Langerhans so that the person is incapable of producing insulin. In type 2 diabetes, the pancreas cannot keep up with the persistent level of hyperglycemia.

167. B: Diverticulosis is the presence of small outpouchings in the colon usually caused by a low-fiber diet. It can be seen on radiologic studies such as CAT scan, but the best diagnostic test is a colonoscopy done by a gastroenterologist.

168. D: Nephrolithiasis is the presence of a kidney stone. Sialolithiasis is the presence of a salivary duct stone. Cholelithiasis is the presence of a gallbladder stone. Choledocholithiasis is the presence of a common bile duct stone. Stones may be asymptomatic and found on routine workup.

169. A: Hepatitis is an infection or inflammation of the liver. Hepat- refers to the liver and the suffix -itis refers to inflammation or infection. It may be due to gallstones viruses, alcohol, drugs, or medications.

170. D: The suffix -pexy means to surgically anchor something to a specific location. If a male child has an undescended testicle, the urologist will perform an orchiopexy. This procedure will prevent the testicle from going back up into the abdominal cavity. Testicles left in the abdominal cavity, known as cryptorchidism, increase the risk of malignancy.

171. B: Cataracts are calcium deposits on the lens of the eye that impair vision. The treatment is a relatively simple surgical removal. The risk of developing cataracts increases with age.

172. C: Cholelithiasis is the presence of stones in the gallbladder. Chole- refers to the gallbladder and the suffix -lithiasis means the presence of stones within a visceral organ. Gallstones do not always have to cause symptoms. They may be found during a routine workup.

173. A: The suffix -rrhagia refers to hemorrhage or excessive flow. For example, menorrhagia is a heavy menstrual period.

174. D: Atrial fibrillation is a cardiac arrhythmia in which the atria do not rhythmically contract. Their activity is unrelated to the contraction of the ventricles. Patients with atrial fibrillation may be asymptomatic or may experience chest pain, shortness of breath, palpitations, or syncope. A cardiologist focuses on structural heart abnormalities and cardiac arrhythmias.

175. C: Oliguria is a low urine output. The prefix oligo- means few or little. The prefix dys- means difficult or painful. The prefix poly- means many. The term hemat refers to blood.

176. D: Sickle cell anemia is an autosomal recessive blood disorder that causes flexible circular red blood cells to be fragile crescent-shaped cells. Since these cells do not flow easily through smaller blood vessels and break down much more easily than normal, patients may have signs and symptoms of ischemia. These episodes are called crises. There is no cure; the goal of treatment is prevention of crises and symptomatic relief.

177. C: A person with a blood pressure of 165/81 mm Hg has hypertension. Hypertension is the medical term for elevated blood pressure. A normal blood pressure for an adult is 120/80 mm Hg. A single elevated blood pressure is not diagnostic of hypertension. There should be several consecutive pressures taken (usually 3 consecutive times spaced a few weeks apart) in order to be given this diagnosis.

178. B: The acetabulum is the hip socket where the femoral head fits into the pelvis. It is a ball and joint socket that allows for people to walk with ease. The risk of injury to this area is higher with babies and elderly individuals.

179. A: Atherosclerosis is the presence of fatty deposits in the medium and large arterial walls. Patients with atherosclerosis may have angina, hypertension, and claudication due to the decreased intraluminal area of the blood vessels. The decreased lumen will restrict blood flow to that area, particularly during activity.

180. A: Schizophrenia is a psychiatric disorder characterized by odd behaviors, hallucinations, impaired social intelligence, reasoning, and emotional instability. Antipsychotic medications may help. A psychiatrist is a physician who specializes in mental disorders.

Practice Test #2

1. According to Maslow's theory of human behavior, what is considered the second-highest level?

    a. Physiological.
    b. Esteem.
    c. Safety.
    d. Social.

2. Which of the following is not a violation of Health Insurance Portability and Accountability Act (HIPAA)?

    a. Releasing patient information to a third party without a patient signature.
    b. Talking about a patient's condition at the nursing desk.
    c. Throwing a medical chart in a trash can.
    d. Discussing a patient's case over social media.

3. When a medical provider asks a patient a question that requires a detailed response, what type of question is he or she asking?

    a. Open.
    b. Investigative.
    c. Direct.
    d. Informative.

4. A person who denies the presence of a negative behavior and blames it on someone else is using what type of defense mechanism?

    a. Regression.
    b. Projection.
    c. Denial.
    d. Displacement.

5. Which level of Maslow's theory of human behavior entails the basic needs for food, water and sleep?

    a. Self-actualization.
    b. Safety.
    c. Esteem.
    d. Physiological.

6. When speaking to someone whose native language is not English, which of the following would not be helpful in communication with the patient?

    a. Having a translator present.
    b. Speaking slowly.
    c. Writing the instructions.
    d. Using hand gestures.

7. A child who is first starting to roll over onto his or her abdomen is likely what age?

  a. 4 to 6 months.
  b. 8 to 10 months.
  c. 12 months.
  d. 18 months.

8. What is the most common first sign of puberty in males?

  a. Enlargement of the testes.
  b. Growth spurt.
  c. Deepening of the voice.
  d. Development of body odor.

9. Which of the following would NOT facilitate communication with a geriatric patient?

  a. Using clear terminology.
  b. Repeating important phrases.
  c. Speaking slowly.
  d. Keeping the voice low.

10. Which of the following is NOT beyond medical assistants' scope of practice?

  a. Prescribing medications.
  b. Taking a patient's vital signs.
  c. Interpreting lab results.
  d. Suturing a laceration.

11. What is the most important piece of information to obtain from a patient when taking a message for a physician?

  a. Birth date.
  b. Name.
  c. Time of the call.
  d. Diagnosis.

12. Typically a male physician examining a female patient should bring which of the following into the examination room?

  a. Camera.
  b. Power of attorney.
  c. Chaperone.
  d. Consent.

13. According to Maslow's theory of human behavior, which of the following levels needs to be fulfilled before progressing to social needs?

  a. Self-actualization and esteem.
  b. Safety and esteem.
  c. Physiological and self-actualization.
  d. Safety and physiological.

14. When is it most appropriate to wash one's hands when examining a patient?

a. Before examining the patient.
b. After examining the patient.
c. Sporadically during the day.
d. Before and after examining the patient.

15. A patient is in the office for a routine well visit. A medical assistant who is pro-life notices a history of an elective abortion on a patient's chart. Which of the following is the MOST appropriate action?

a. Hand the patient a pro-life brochure.
b. Refuse to see the patient.
c. Lecture the patient on the dangers of abortion.
d. Inquire if the patient had any post-procedure complications.

16. A medical assistant comes into the office in the morning. He notices that an urgent message left by a patient last night needs to be returned, paperwork needs to be filed, a patient is at the desk with a question, and a lab tray needs to be set up for an appointment in an hour. Which of the following tasks should be completed first?

a. Addressing the telephone message.
b. Filing paperwork.
c. Addressing the patient at the desk.
d. Setting up the lab tray.

17. A woman comes to the office for a routine well visit. She is devoutly religious and requests that she not be examined by a medical assistant or a physician of the opposite sex. Which of the following is the MOST appropriate response?

a. Request that she go to another office.
b. Compromise by bringing in a female chaperone.
c. Have a female medical assistant and physician see the patient.
d. Have a male medical provider examine her anyway.

18. According to Maslow's theory of human behavior, which of the following should be fulfilled before progressing to safety needs?

a. Achievement.
b. Shelter.
c. Friendship.
d. Personal growth.

19. Which of the following mannerisms would be least likely to be considered hostile or aggressive?

a. Low voice.
b. Close proximity.
c. Expressionless face.
d. Sudden movements and gestures.

20. Which of the following would NOT aid a visually impaired patient?

    a. Providing a brightly lit room.
    b. Using large block lettering.
    c. Speaking in a loud voice.
    d. Holding his or her arm when ambulating.

21. A child who is starting to walk without assistance is most likely what age?

    a. 6 months.
    b. 12 months.
    c. 18 months.
    d. 24 months.

22. A patient has just been diagnosed with stage IV breast cancer. Her son offers the physician money and orders the physician to save her life. What stage of grief is the son in according to Kübler-Ross?

    a. Anger.
    b. Acceptance.
    c. Denial.
    d. Bargaining.

23. Which of the following is TRUE regarding the Genetic Information Nondiscrimination Act of 2008?

    a. It prevents insurers from discriminating against people based on genetic information.
    b. It ensures schools provide necessary accommodations to those with preexisting conditions.
    c. It prevents employers from discriminating against people based on genetic information.
    d. It ensures restaurants and businesses provide necessary accommodations to those with preexisting conditions.

24. When a medical provider asks a patient a question that requires a one-word response, what type of question is he or she asking?

    a. Open.
    b. Investigative.
    c. Direct.
    d. Informative.

25. According to Maslow's theory of human behavior, which of the following does NOT describe someone who has achieved self-actualization?

    a. Creative.
    b. Spontaneous.
    c. Self-centered.
    d. Open to new experiences.

26. Four patients arrive in the emergency room at the same time: a patient with a gunshot wound to the arm, a patient who is seizing, a patient with an asthma exacerbation, and a patient with a dislocated shoulder. Which patient should be addressed last?

    a. Gunshot wound.
    b. Seizure.
    c. Asthma exacerbation.
    d. Shoulder dislocation.

27. Which of the following is FALSE regarding Occupational Safety and Health Administration (OSHA)?

    a. Employers must inform workers of work hazards through training.
    b. Employers must protect employees from discrimination if they report work hazards.
    c. Employers must provide employees with free personal protective gear.
    d. Employers must provide employees with job benefits and vacation time.

28. Which of the following practices is prohibited by the Fair Debt Collection Practices Act (FDCPA)?

    a. Calling a consumer after a consumer verbally requests the calls to cease.
    b. Calling a consumer at 4 a.m.
    c. Contacting a consumer's attorney.
    d. Contacting the consumer's spouse regarding the debt owed.

29. A 5-year-old patient is brought to the emergency room with a broken wrist and bruising clusters on both arms. What is the MOST appropriate initial response?

    a. Chide the child about being more careful around hot water.
    b. Order X-rays of the hands and feet.
    c. Call child protective services.
    d. Refer the patient to a dermatologist.

30. What is the medical term for a woman's first period?

    a. Menopause.
    b. Menses.
    c. Menorrhagia.
    d. Menarche.

31. A patient is a suspected victim of domestic abuse. Which of the following questions is the MOST inappropriate?

    a. How do you and your partner relate to each other?
    b. Have you ever been concerned about your safety or that of your children?
    c. Why do you allow yourself to be abused?
    d. Is everything alright at home?

32. Which of the following is not communicated by respiratory droplets?

    a. Tuberculosis.
    b. Hepatitis B.
    c. Influenza.
    d. Croup.

33. Which of the following is a violation of Health Insurance Portability and Accountability Act (HIPAA)?

    a. Discussing the patient's prognosis with his or her power of attorney.
    b. Sending a patient's records to his or her designated primary care doctor.
    c. Keeping yourself logged into the hospital computer to allow quicker documentation.
    d. Disposing of sensitive documents in a shredder.

34. Which of the following best describes universal precautions?

a. Treating human body fluids as if they contained infectious diseases.
b. Medical precautions taken when traveling abroad.
c. Ensuring the vaccination of all children.
d. The use of prophylactic medications.

35. Which of the following is the LEAST important piece of information when taking an urgent message?

a. Time of call.
b. Telephone number.
c. Address.
d. Name.

36. Which of the following is NOT a venereal disease?

a. HIV.
b. Varicella.
c. Chlamydia.
d. Syphilis.

37. Which of the following statements regarding the Truth in Lending Act (TILA) of 1968 is MOST accurate?

a. TILA limits the amount of interest that may be charged.
b. It mandates that the annual percentage rate (APR) must be disclosed to the consumer.
c. TILA regulates the amount of fees that consumers can be charged for late payments.
d. It mandates businesses to work with consumers who have poor credit.

38. Which medication is the LEAST likely to be investigated by the Drug Enforcement Agency (DEA)?

a. Oxycodone.
b. Pseudoephedrine.
c. Morphine sulfate.
d. Amoxicillin.

39. Which of the following conditions is the MOST dangerous?

a. Croup.
b. Ankle fracture.
c. Third-degree burn.
d. Conjunctivitis.

40. What is the MOST common blood-borne illness in the United States?

a. Roseola.
b. AIDS.
c. Varicella.
d. Hepatitis C.

41. Which of the following classes of medications would NOT be controlled by the Drug Enforcement Agency (DEA)?

a. Antibiotics.
b. Antipsychotics.
c. Benzodiazepines.
d. Narcotics.

42. Which of the following is NOT a function of the Center for Disease Control (CDC)?

a. Identifies national and international health threats.
b. Regulates and supervises vaccines.
c. Develops laboratory guidelines.
d. Promotes healthy behaviors and practices.

43. What bodily fluid has the highest risk for transmitting HIV/AIDS?

a. Saliva.
b. Feces.
c. Urine.
d. Semen.

44. Which situation is the best example of implied consent?

a. Rolling up a sleeve for a blood pressure check.
b. Signing paperwork agreeing to a surgery.
c. Nodding in the affirmative prior to a procedure.
d. Verbalizing one's comprehension of the risks and benefits of treatment.

45. What is the best statement that describes an emancipated minor?

a. A person who is freed from control of their parents.
b. Someone who is charged with a crime in their childhood.
c. A person who is adopted in young adulthood.
d. Someone who cannot make his or her own medical decisions.

46. All of the following are within a medical assistant's scope of practice EXCEPT:

a. scheduling patient appointments.
b. performing laceration repair.
c. documenting vital signs.
d. administering electrocardiograms.

47. Which of the following describes the ability to make one's own medical decisions?

a. Tort.
b. Capacity.
c. Living will.
d. Deposition.

48. Which of the following is a function of the Food and Drug Administration (FDA)?

a. Sets drug prices.
b. Regulates dietary supplements.
c. Creates vaccines for emerging illnesses.
d. Develops new prescription drugs.

49. What is the legal term requiring a patient to appear in court to provide certain documentation?

a. Locum tenens.
b. Subpoena duces tecum.
c. Arbitration.
d. Res ipsa loquitor.

50. A physician prescribes a medication to a patient who develops an anaphylactic reaction and subsequently dies. It is documented in the patient's chart that he or she was allergic to this medication. What type of crime did the physician commit?

a. Assault.
b. Slander.
c. Negligence.
d. Libel.

51. According to Erikson's stages of development, which of the following conflicts would not take place during school-age years?

a. Initiative versus guilt.
b. Industry versus inferiority.
c. Identity versus confusion.
d. Generativity versus stagnation.

52. Which of the following would be the LEAST helpful when trying to communicate with someone who speaks little English?

a. Having a staff member translate.
b. Ensuring that an English-speaking family member or friend is present.
c. Speaking slowly in a loud voice.
d. Having consent forms that are in the patient's native language.

53. A patient calls the office demanding to speak to the physician immediately regarding an urgent issue. What is the MOST important initial question to ask the patient?

a. What is the issue regarding?
b. When did you last come to the office for a visit?
c. Can you call back later when the physician isn't busy?
d. What is your insurance plan?

54. A physician is accused of molesting a patient while she was under anesthesia. What crime did the physician allegedly commit?

a. Negligence.
b. Theft.
c. Assault.
d. Perjury.

55. An elderly patient with known history of mild Alzheimer's disease gives a $50 bill for her $20 copay. What is the MOST appropriate action?

a. Give the woman $30.
b. Take the extra money, and donate it to Alzheimer's research.
c. Put the extra money in the office's petty cash.
d. Buy the office staff lunch.

56. A woman is diagnosed with chlamydia. What should she be advised to do next?

a. Continue having unprotected sex because she has been treated.
b. Don't tell anyone about the diagnosis because it may ruin her reputation.
c. Once she has contracted the disease, she will have immunity to it.
d. Call previous partners, and inform them of her diagnosis.

57. A child is brought to the hospital by his father with a concussion and fractured arm. This is the second episode. What is the MOST appropriate initial action?

a. Blame the mother.
b. Call an orthopedist.
c. Call Child Protective Services.
d. Blame the father.

58. A patient has a history of verbally abusing the office staff and the physician. The patient has a complicated medical history that requires frequent office visits. What can be done about this patient?

a. Send the patient to the emergency room for medical care.
b. Terminate the patient-physician relationship.
c. Try and have the patient arrested.
d. Refuse to schedule appointments for the patient.

59. Which of the following measures may help prevent workplace accidents?

a. Dim lighting.
b. Carpeting.
c. Non-adjustable equipment.
d. Tile floors.

60. What is the Latin phrase that means "without negligence the accident would not have happened"?

a. Per diem.
b. Respondeat superior.
c. Carpe diem.
d. Res ipsa loquitur.

61. A patient's sister states that she is a physician and requests to see her sister's medical records regarding her condition. What is the MOST appropriate action?

a. Refuse to let the sister see the medical records under any condition.
b. Call the police, and accuse the patient's sister of libel.
c. Check the woman's ID before giving her the medical records.
d. Tell the patient consent must be signed authorizing her sister to view the records.

62. A medical assistant witnesses a nurse administer the incorrect medication to a patient. There are no negative sequelae from this event. What should the medical assistant do?

a. Do not report the incident because nothing happened to the patient.
b. Threaten to fire the nurse.
c. Report the incident to administration.
d. Announce the event on social media.

63. What is the medical term for surgically rerouting the large intestine through an opening in the abdominal wall?

a. Colostomy.
b. Gastrectomy.
c. Urostomy.
d. Colectomy.

64. What does the suffix -itis mean?

a. Presence of.
b. Inflammation.
c. Surgical repair.
d. Hemorrhage.

65. Which of the following represents structures in the arm?

a. Ulna, radius, olecranon.
b. Ulna, tibia, phalange.
c. Femur, tibia, fibula.
d. Fibula, humerus, sternum.

66. What is the medical term for ankle?

a. Phalange.
b. Patella.
c. Malleolus.
d. Scapula.

67. Which of the following is superior to the acetabulum?

a. Axilla.
b. Spleen.
c. Clavicle.
d. Patella.

68. What does the suffix -acusis mean?

a. Vision.
b. Pain.
c. Malodorous.
d. Hearing.

69. A medical assistant is caring for a patient who has suffered a stroke. He overhears the physician say that the patient is aphasic. What type of deficit does this patient have?

a. Inability to move a part of the body.
b. Trouble swallowing.
c. Difficulty with speech.
d. Inability to walk.

70. A patient with cervical cancer should be referred to which specialist?

a. Hematologist.
b. Gynecologist.
c. Gastroenterologist.
d. Rheumatologist.

71. **Which of the following should be worn at all times when doing procedures?**

    a. Eye goggles.
    b. Gown.
    c. Gloves.
    d. Mask.

72. **Which of the following subjects should NOT be on office memos?**

    a. Arguments among staff.
    b. Maintenance regulations.
    c. Safety protocols.
    d. Schedules.

73. **A patient has a torn meniscus. Which type of procedure is needed?**

    a. Lithotripsy.
    b. Hemorrhoidectomy.
    c. Sigmoidoscopy.
    d. Arthroscopy.

74. **What is the term for the method of keeping track of office supplies?**

    a. Encryption.
    b. Inventory.
    c. Diagnostics.
    d. Itemized statements.

75. **What is the medical term for breastplate?**

    a. Clavicle.
    b. Sternum.
    c. Scapula.
    d. Epicondyle.

76. **When would it be MOST appropriate to first send an unpaid bill to a collection agency?**

    a. Three days.
    b. Three weeks.
    c. Three months.
    d. Three years.

77. **A patient with Crohn's disease should be referred to which specialist?**

    a. Gastroenterologist.
    b. Urologist.
    c. Orthopedist.
    d. Psychiatrist.

78. **Which of the following represents structures in the abdominal cavity?**

    a. Kidneys, duodenum, bladder, stomach.
    b. Pancreas, meniscus, spleen, kidneys.
    c. Liver, adrenals, stomach, acetabulum.
    d. Ureter, gallbladder, liver, duodenum.

79. **Which of the following is the MOST appropriate use of petty cash?**

    a. Cell phones.
    b. Take-out.
    c. Manila folders.
    d. Cab fare.

80. **A patient with psoriasis should be referred to which specialist?**

    a. Cardiologist.
    b. Psychiatrist.
    c. Dermatologist.
    d. Urologist.

81. **Which of the following people would not be eligible for the Civilian Health and Medical Program of the Department of Veterans Affairs (CHAMPVA)?**

    a. An unmarried ex-spouse of a permanently disabled veteran.
    b. A spouse who died of a veteran-related disability.
    c. A child of a permanently disabled veteran.
    d. A child of a disabled veteran released from service for misconduct.

82. **Which of the following patients is MOST appropriate for Tricare?**

    a. A mentally disabled child.
    b. A patient with a very low income.
    c. An elderly patient.
    d. A marine.

83. **Which of the following structures are not inside the thoracic cavity?**

    a. Lungs.
    b. Trachea.
    c. Heart.
    d. Duodenum.

84. **What structure is lateral to the liver?**

    a. Bladder.
    b. Kidneys.
    c. Spleen.
    d. Gallbladder.

85. **What structure is ventral to the lungs?**

    a. Sternum.
    b. Trachea.
    c. Diaphragm.
    d. Spine.

86. **Which of the following pairs is separated by a transverse plane?**

    a. Right and left arms.
    b. Head and feet.
    c. Sternum and the spine.
    d. Right and left legs.

87. **Where is the malleolus in relation to the femur?**

    a. Inferior.
    b. Anterior.
    c. Posterior.
    d. Dorsal.

88. **What structure is NOT inferior to the kidney?**

    a. Adrenal gland.
    b. Sigmoid colon.
    c. Appendix.
    d. Cervix.

89. **Which system provides support and movement to the body?**

    a. Integumentary.
    b. Musculoskeletal.
    c. Nervous.
    d. Endocrine.

90. **How many stages are in the chain of infection?**

    a. Two.
    b. Four.
    c. Six.
    d. Eight.

91. **Which of the following would be considered the best type of susceptible host for infection to spread?**

    a. A patient with a fractured humerus.
    b. A patient with dementia.
    c. A patient with Hodgkin's lymphoma.
    d. A patient with glaucoma.

92. **Which system would be MOST affected by pyelonephritis?**

    a. Reproductive.
    b. Gastrointestinal.
    c. Nervous.
    d. Urinary.

93. **What organism needs a host to survive?**

    a. Bacteria.
    b. Mitochondria.
    c. Nucleus.
    d. Parasite.

94. **Which of the following is NOT a shared characteristic between viruses and bacteria?**

    a. They contain cell walls.
    b. They contain DNA or RNA.
    c. They lack a nucleus.
    d. They contain enzymes.

95. A mistake is made while writing a progress note. What is the MOST appropriate course of action?

a. Use white out.
b. Cross out the error once and initial it.
c. Throw out the note and start over.
d. Scribble out the mistake and keep writing.

96. Where are the mammary glands in relation to the spine?

a. Contralateral.
b. Ventral.
c. Ipsilateral.
d. Dorsal.

97. Which represents a normal heart rate in an adult human?

a. 20 beats per minute.
b. 60 beats per minute.
c. 120 beats per minute.
d. 160 beats per minute.

98. Where is the appendix located in a nonpregnant person with typical anatomy?

a. Left lower quadrant.
b. Right upper quadrant.
c. Left upper quadrant.
d. Right lower quadrant.

99. Which represents a normal pulse oximetry reading on room air?

a. 100 percent.
b. 90 percent.
c. 75 percent.
d. 50 percent.

100. Which system would be most affected by leukemia?

a. Hematologic.
b. Nervous.
c. Cardiopulmonary.
d. Genitourinary.

101. In regard to the chain of infection, which would NOT be a portal of entry?

a. Ingestion.
b. Inhalation.
c. Perspiration.
d. Penetration.

102. What is NOT a likely location for pulse oximeter placement?

a. Fingertip.
b. Sublingual.
c. Earlobe.
d. Toe.

103. What is the average body temperature in a human (in Fahrenheit)?

a. 96.8 degrees.
b. 100 degrees.
c. 98.6 degrees.
d. 37 degrees.

104. What is a common spot to palpate a pulse during a routine office visit?

a. Popliteal artery.
b. Dorsalis pedis artery.
c. Radial artery.
d. Femoral artery.

105. Which system would be MOST affected by celiac disease?

a. Integumentary.
b. Gastrointestinal.
c. Reproductive.
d. Endocrine.

106. Which of the following statements belongs in the chief complaint section of a progress note?

a. Abdominal pain for five days.
b. Employed as a lawyer.
c. Tylenol helping to alleviate pain.
d. History of alcohol abuse.

107. Fungi would commonly be found in which location?

a. Water.
b. Semen.
c. Blood.
d. Mold.

108. In regard to the chain of infection, which best represents a reservoir?

a. Virus.
b. Soil.
c. Quarantine.
d. Hand washing.

109. Which of the following items should be sterilized in an autoclave?

a. Colonoscope.
b. Holter monitor.
c. Syringe.
d. Sphygmomanometer.

110. Which system would be MOST affected by endometriosis?

a. Nervous.
b. Endocrine.
c. Reproductive.
d. Cardiopulmonary.

111. What position is a patient in when he or she is lying facedown?

a. Lateral recumbent.
b. Trendelenberg.
c. Supine.
d. Prone.

112. At what age should MOST patients get their first colonoscopy?

a. 30 years old.
b. 40 years old.
c. 50 years old.
d. 60 years old.

113. How often should a woman perform a breast exam?

a. Daily.
b. Weekly.
c. Monthly.
d. Yearly.

114. What position is a patient in when he or she is lying flat on his or her back with his or her head tilted downward?

a. Trendelenberg.
b. Reverse Trendelenberg.
c. Fowlers.
d. Lithotomy.

115. A patient with hypertension should limit which of the following?

a. Chloride.
b. Glucose.
c. Magnesium.
d. Sodium.

116. Which of the following laboratory values evaluates blood viscosity?

a. Erythrocyte sedimentation rate.
b. White blood cell count.
c. Hematocrit.
d. International normalized ratio.

117. Which of the following lab values monitors kidney function?

a. Creatinine.
b. Low density lipoprotein.
c. Hemoglobin A1C.
d. Thyroxine.

118. A patient with celiac disease should avoid which of the following?

a. Peanuts.
b. Crackers.
c. Milk.
d. Candy.

119. H. pylori is responsible for which of the following?

    a. Endometriosis.
    b. Cervical cancer.
    c. Gastritis.
    d. Otitis media.

120. Which of the following should be limited or avoided in a patient with lactose intolerance?

    a. Spinach.
    b. Cheese.
    c. Strawberries.
    d. Red meat.

121. A patient's occupation should be in which section of the progress note?

    a. Physical exam.
    b. Chief complaint.
    c. Social history.
    d. History of present illness.

122. When is the best time for a patient's blood pressure to be taken during an office visit?

    a. As soon as they arrive.
    b. While giving them unpleasant news.
    c. After sitting in a chair for several minutes.
    d. When getting undressed for an exam.

123. Which of the following is a normal respiratory rate in a healthy adult?

    a. 6 breaths per minute.
    b. 16 breaths per minute.
    c. 26 breaths per minute.
    d. 36 breaths per minute.

124. Which of the following is NOT needed for suture removal?

    a. Scissors.
    b. Skin glue.
    c. Band-Aid.
    d. Gloves.

125. Which of the following is the best technique for prepping the skin prior to a procedure?

    a. Make gradually enlarging circles around the future incision site.
    b. Make a criss-cross pattern.
    c. Shake the prep onto the body, making a splatter pattern.
    d. Make a zigzag pattern.

126. Through which route is insulin administered?

    a. Rectal.
    b. Oral.
    c. Intramuscular.
    d. Subcutaneous.

127. A poorly controlled diabetic patient should be advised to check his or her sugars at what intervals during the day?

　　a. After meals and in the morning.
　　b. Before meals and at bedtime.
　　c. After meals only.
　　d. At bedtime only.

128. Which of the following is NOT a direct cause of tobacco use?

　　a. Myocardial infarction.
　　b. Diabetes.
　　c. Chronic bronchitis.
　　d. Malignancy.

129. Through which route is the influenza vaccine usually administered?

　　a. Rectal.
　　b. Subcutaneous.
　　c. Intramuscular.
　　d. Intravenous.

130. How often should women have Pap smears?

　　a. Weekly.
　　b. Monthly.
　　c. Yearly.
　　d. Every 10 years.

131. Which of the following should receive the pneumococcal vaccination?

　　a. A patient status post kidney transplant.
　　b. An AIDS patient.
　　c. A patient with multiple myeloma.
　　d. A patient with diabetes.

132. What type of fracture involves a bend and crack of the bone?

　　a. Colles.
　　b. Greenstick.
　　c. Oblique.
　　d. Transverse.

133. What is the MOST common type of stroke?

　　a. Ischemic.
　　b. Hemorrhagic.
　　c. Subdural.
　　d. Subarachnoid.

134. Which of the following is NOT a treatment for poisoning?

　　a. Gastric lavage.
　　b. Whole bowel irrigation.
　　c. Antivenom.
　　d. Antibiotics.

135. Which of the following best describes an absence seizure?

   a. Blank staring.
   b. Generalized tremors.
   c. Syncope.
   d. Hemiparesis.

136. What is the treatment for diabetic ketoacidosis?

   a. Insulin.
   b. Sugar.
   c. Antibiotics.
   d. Antivirals.

137. Which best defines an oblique fracture?

   a. A diagonal fracture.
   b. Separation from a joint.
   c. A horizontal fracture.
   d. Splintering into several pieces.

138. A right-sided stroke will MOST likely affect which part of the body?

   a. Left arm.
   b. Vision.
   c. Right arm.
   d. Digestion.

139. What radiological study is the best choice to evaluate a joint dislocation?

   a. X-ray.
   b. PET scan.
   c. MRI.
   d. CAT scan.

140. What is the medical term for passing out?

   a. Tinnitus.
   b. Vertigo.
   c. Syncope.
   d. Hemiparesis.

141. What is the medical term for gait dysfunction?

   a. Aphagia.
   b. Apraxia.
   c. Aphasia.
   d. Ataxia.

142. What is the medical term for an abnormal, high-pitched rattling or whistling sound made while breathing?

   a. Murmur.
   b. Wheezing.
   c. Seizure.
   d. Dysphagia.

143. Which of the following would be treated by an automated external defibrillator?

a. Tachycardia.
b. Asystole.
c. Bradycardia.
d. Ventricular fibrillation.

144. Which of the following best describes a grand mal seizure?

a. Generalized tremors.
b. Blank staring.
c. Incontinence.
d. Drooling.

145. If there is a question regarding a vaccine's expiration date, what would be the MOST appropriate action?

a. Keep it in the refrigerator.
b. Use it immediately.
c. Throw it away.
d. Mix it with another vaccine with a later expiration date.

146. Which of following best describes a simple partial seizure?

a. Nausea.
b. Vision changes.
c. Focal tremors.
d. Loss of consciousness.

147. Which of the following is not part of the six rights of medication administration?

a. Right patient.
b. Right consent.
c. Right dose.
d. Right route.

148. Which of the following is NOT a severe complication of hemorrhage?

a. Hypoxia.
b. Heart attack.
c. Syncope.
d. Diabetes insipidus.

149. What is the medical term for a respiratory rate of 32 breaths per minute?

a. Bradycardia.
b. Tachypnea.
c. Tachycardia.
d. Bradypnea.

150. A medication needs to be taken under the tongue. What is the medical term for this type of administration?

a. Sublingual.
b. Intradermal.
c. Oral.
d. Subcutaneous.

151. All of the following items are typically found in a crash cart EXCEPT:

    a. a stethoscope.
    b. a laryngoscope.
    c. syringes.
    d. alcohol swabs.

152. Which of the following is the MOST severe type of drug reaction?

    a. Hives.
    b. Pruritus.
    c. Nausea.
    d. Anaphylaxis.

153. Which of the following is the best way to assess responsiveness of a patient?

    a. Pour cold water on his or her face.
    b. Hit him or her.
    c. Tap on his or her chest, and ask if he or she is awake.
    d. Listen to his or her heart.

154. What is the MOST common concern with feral animal bites?

    a. Diphtheria.
    b. Rabies.
    c. Polio.
    d. AIDS.

155. According to advanced cardiac life support (ACLS) protocol, how many chest compressions should be performed in a minute?

    a. 50.
    b. 100.
    c. 150.
    d. 200.

156. Where is the best location to assess a pulse in an unresponsive patient?

    a. Dorsalis pedis.
    b. Carotid.
    c. Radial.
    d. Popliteal.

157. Which of the following is NOT a symptom of vertigo?

    a. Vomiting.
    b. Nausea.
    c. Seizure.
    d. Dizziness.

158. When should a person stop administering the Heimlich maneuver?

    a. When the person administering the maneuver gets tired.
    b. When the person starts turning blue.
    c. When a rib is broken.
    d. When a patient becomes unconscious.

159. Which of the following medications can be safely used during pregnancy?

a. Pregnancy category B.
b. Pregnancy category C.
c. Pregnancy category F.
d. Pregnancy category A.

160. Who can do cardiopulmonary resuscitation (CPR)?

a. Physicians.
b. Nurses.
c. Medical Assistants.
d. Anyone who has passed a certification course.

161. Which of the following evaluates for potential dermal allergic reactions?

a. Rinne test.
b. Pulmonary function test.
c. Scratch test.
d. Weber test.

162. A woman's serum beta hcg is 52 mIU/ml three days after her expected menses. Two days later it is rechecked, and the result is 85 mIU/ml. What can be said about the status of this pregnancy?

a. Impending miscarriage.
b. Unknown.
c. Ectopic.
d. Normal pregnancy.

163. Which of the following labs helps monitor inflammation?

a. Erythrocyte sedimentation rate (ESR).
b. Blood urea nitrogen (BUN).
c. Creatinine phosphokinase (CPK).
d. Hemoglobin A1c (HA1c).

164. An Epstein-Barr virus (EBV) causes which of the following diseases?

a. Influenza.
b. Pneumonia.
c. Mononucleosis.
d. AIDS.

165. Spontaneous bleeding is caused by which of the following conditions?

a. Leukocytosis.
b. Thrombocytopenia.
c. Leukopenia.
d. Thrombocytosis.

166. Of the choices given, what is the MOST common method for evaluating potential dermal allergic reactions?

    a. Intradermal.
    b. Intramuscular.
    c. Oral.
    d. Rectal.

167. Which of the following means to adjust a measuring device?

    a. Catheterization.
    b. Centrifuge.
    c. Cardiovert.
    d. Calibration.

168. Which of the following means to preserve or stabilize something?

    a. Fragmentation.
    b. Fixative.
    c. Ferment.
    d. Fluoroscopy.

169. Where would the corpus callosum be located?

    a. Liver.
    b. Heart.
    c. Brain.
    d. Lung.

170. Which test is used to identify hearing threshold levels?

    a. Weber test.
    b. Cold caloric test.
    c. Pure tone audiometry.
    d. Rinne test.

171. In a 12-lead electrocardiogram (ECG) how many precordial chest leads are there?

    a. Two.
    b. Four.
    c. Six.
    d. Eight.

172. What is the primary purpose of a Holter monitor?

    a. Evaluate for vegetation.
    b. Diagnose heart attacks.
    c. Evaluate for arrhythmias.
    d. Determine ejection fraction.

173. A heart rate of 125 beats per minute with absent or irregular p-waves best describes which of the following arrhythmias?

    a. Supraventricular tachycardia.
    b. Asystole.
    c. Atrial fibrillation.
    d. First-degree heart block.

174. What part of the heart acts as a "back-up pacemaker"?

a. Purkinje fibers.
b. Sinus node.
c. Foramen ovale.
d. Atrioventricular node.

175. Which of the following reflects a normal QRS complex?

a. 0.08 seconds.
b. 0.80 seconds.
c. 2.0 seconds.
d. 0.20 seconds.

176. Which of the following cannot be detected by a 12-lead EKG?

a. Rhythm.
b. Ischemia.
c. Vegetation.
d. Rate.

177. Which of the following reflects a PR interval seen with first degree heart block?

a. 0.012.
b. 0.016.
c. 0.020.
d. 0.024.

178. A Jaeger card is used to assess which of the following?

a. Gait.
b. Hearing.
c. Speech.
d. Vision.

179. Increased ocular pressure is seen with which of the following pathologies?

a. Macular degeneration.
b. Glaucoma.
c. Cataracts.
d. Corneal abrasion.

180. Which of the following best describes first-degree heart block?

a. A constant prolonged PR interval.
b. No association between p-waves and QRS complexes.
c. An increasing PR interval with intermittent dropped p-waves.
d. A sawtooth pattern.

Answers and Explanations

1. B: Food, water, sleep, and excretion are the four fundamental needs according to Maslow's Hierarchy. These needs have to be fulfilled for a person to have a sense of peace and safety. The next level includes security of oneself and the safety of loved ones. The next level includes fulfillment of relationships with family members and friends and intimacy with loved ones. Self-esteem is the second-highest level, followed by the highest level of self-actualization.

2. B: Talking about a case in voices at a reasonable volume is not a HIPAA violation. Taking about a case in public areas such as elevators or cafeterias would be a violation of patient privacy. Releasing medical information without consent, throwing away a chart in a non-designated trash bin, or talking about a case on social media are also violations.

3. A: There are two types of questions: open and direct. An open-ended question requires an answer with some detailed explanation or depth. A closed or a direct question requires only one-word answers such as yes or no.

4. B: Projection is a type of defense mechanism where a person displays a negative behavior and blames it on someone else. For example, a woman may accuse her significant other of cheating, but she is the one who is unfaithful.

5. D: Food, water, sleep, and excretion are the four fundamental needs according to Maslow's Hierarchy. These needs have to be fulfilled for a person to have a sense of peace and safety. These needs also allow the individual to fulfill the subsequent needs in Maslow's hierarchy.

6. C: If a patient speaks little or no English, chances are he or she will not be able to read it either. Speaking slowly so that the translator receives all of the information being given, using hand gestures, or drawing pictures may help facilitate communication.

7. A: Although ages at which developmental milestones are reached vary among children, generally children start rolling over onto their abdomen at 4 to 6 months. At 8 to 12 months children start crawling, at 12 months they may start to walk, and by 18 months they can run without much difficulty.

8. A: There are many signs at the onset of puberty, such as the growth of hair on the face, axilla, chest, and testes; deepening of the voice; development of body odor; and growth spurts. The most common initial sign is enlargement of the testes.

9. D: Keeping one's voice low would not help facilitate communication in an elderly patient. Most elderly patients have hearing difficulties. When speaking to the elderly, one should speak in a loud, clear, slow voice so that no information is missed.

10. B: Medical assistants have many responsibilities, such as taking vital signs, filing medical records, corresponding with insurances companies, as well as administrative duties. They cannot prescribe medications, interpret labs or radiological scans, insert IVs or catheters, or suture.

11. B: The patient's name is the most important piece of information when taking a message. The time of call, diagnosis, and the birth date are helpful but not necessarily mandatory.

12. C: A chaperone should be utilized when doing an exam on a patient. A chaperone should be always present, especially if a gynecological, rectal, or urological exam is being performed.

13. D: Food, water, sleep, and excretion are the four fundamental needs according to Maslow's Hierarchy. These needs have to be fulfilled for a person to have a sense of peace and safety. The next level includes security of oneself and the safety of loved ones. The next level includes fulfillment of relationships with family members and friends and intimacy with loved ones. Self-esteem is the second-highest level, followed by the highest level of self-actualization.

14. D: Hand washing is the number one way to help prevent the spread of diseases. Medical practitioners should wash their hands before and after examining every patient; after touching keyboards, or equipment; and handling bodily fluids.

15. D: Medical practitioners are allowed to have their own beliefs and opinions but should not impose those beliefs on their patients. Patients should all be given the same respect despite their religion, race, gender, sexual orientation, beliefs regarding abortion, or political views.

16. A: The urgent telephone message should be addressed first. After that task has been addressed, assistance can be provided to the patient at the desk. The lab tray should be set up for the upcoming appointment. Filing paperwork can be done last.

17. C: The patient's wishes are reasonable and should be accommodated. If the situation was life-threatening and only a medical provider of the opposite sex was available, then the patient's request may not be a priority.

18. B: Food, water, sleep, and excretion are the four fundamental needs according to Maslow's Hierarchy. These needs have to be fulfilled for a person to have a sense of peace and safety. The next level includes security of oneself and the safety of loved ones. The next level includes fulfillment of relationships with family members and friends and intimacy with loved ones. Self-esteem is the second-highest level, followed by the highest level of self-actualization.

19. A: Using a low, soothing voice would help communicate nonaggressive intentions. Close proximity can be misconstrued as aggression. An expressionless face can be misunderstood as aggression or apathy. Sudden movements and gestures may relay the message of being upset or angry.

20. C: The patient is visually impaired, not deaf. Talking in a loud voice will not help convey the message. A brightly lit room may help the patient see a little better and prevent accidental falls. Using large, clear, block-print lettering will help him or her read a little better. Holding his or her arm while ambulating may also help prevent falls.

21. B: There is a wide age range in which babies may begin walking. Some may start at 9 months, whereas others may not walk until well after a year. On average children generally start walking around 1 year of age.

22. D: Bargaining with God, a medical professional, or someone with perceived authority as an attempt to save oneself or a loved one is the third stage of grief according to Kubler-Ross. Bargaining can be manifested by financial offers, desperate prayers, or promises in exchange for the desired outcome. The five stages include denial, anger, bargaining, depression, and acceptance.

23. A: The Genetic Information Nondiscrimination Act (GINA) allows people to obtain medical insurance without being discriminated against by companies for preexisting conditions. For example, if someone has sickle cell disease, his or her health care costs will be far higher than those without the disease. If someone has the sickle cell trait, he or she does not have the disease but is capable of passing it to his or her offspring. In the event his or her offspring has sickle cell disease, the health care costs will be high.

24. C: There are two types of questions: open and direct. An open-ended question requires an answer with some detailed explanation or depth. A closed or a direct question requires only one-word answers such as yes or no.

25. C: According to Maslow, people who achieve self-actualization are intelligent, curious, creative, multitalented, and independent and show empathy toward others.

26. D: Patients should always be triaged in terms of severity of their conditions and the potential for their conditions to be life-threatening. A patient who is actively seizing should be cared for first. The seizure needs to be stopped, and the airway needs to be maintained. A gunshot wound to the arm needs to be addressed next to make sure that the bleeding is controlled and the patient is neurovascularly intact. An asthma exacerbation should be addressed next to ensure airway competency. Last to be addressed is the shoulder dislocation. It may be painful but is not dangerous.

27. D: The Occupational Safety and Health Administration's (OSHA's) job is to ensure safety in the workplace. It requires the employer to provide free, functioning safety gear, open disclosure about potential work hazards, and a system of reporting lapses in safety. OSHA does not address job benefits and vacation time.

28. B: The Fair Debt Collection Practices Act (FDCPA) prohibits harassment of customers by debt collectors. Calling a customer outside regular business hours is considered harassment. A customer must state in writing that she or he is in the process of resolving his or her debt for the collector to stop calling. The collector may continue to call unless the request is put in writing. The collector may contact the customer's attorney to discuss the case. The collector may call a spouse regarding the debt owed but is not allowed to call friends, neighbors, and employers.

29. C: A child with a history of extremity fractures or bruising patterns may be a victim of abuse. The medical provider should not approach the family on his or her own; the Division of Family and Youth Services (DYFS) or Child Protective Services (CPS) should be called to investigate further. An orthopedist may be called to evaluate the patient's wrist, but CPS should be notified immediately.

30. D: Menarche is the medical term for the onset of menses. It usually occurs in a woman's early teens, although it may occur even earlier. The cessation of a woman's menses is called menopause. It usually occurs in the fourth or fifth decade of life.

31. C: Using a condescending or angry tone of voice or placing blame on the patient is not appropriate. The patient will not talk to a provider about sensitive issues such as abuse if he or she feels that he or she is being judged or blamed. The patient may become angry, especially if there is no ongoing abuse in the home. When talking to a patient about suspected abuse, the best approach is to ask open-ended questions regarding his or her health and feelings of safety in the home.

32. B: Hepatitis B is an infection of the liver that is transmitted via blood or semen. Tuberculosis, influenza, and croup are respiratory diseases spread via droplets.

33. C: Not logging off a computer properly exposes patients' sensitive information to others. Discussing the case with someone other than a patient's designated representative, sending patient records to physicians not directly involved in the patient's care, and improperly disposing of sensitive documents are other forms of HIPAA violations.

34. A: Universal precautions dictate that medical providers treat all patients and bodily fluids as if they had communicable diseases. Preventative measures such as gloves and consistent hand washing should be done at all times.

35. C: When taking an urgent message, the patient's name, brief summary of the issue, contact information, and time of call should be documented. An address could be helpful but is generally not warranted.

36. B: Varicella, also known as the chicken pox, is a viral infection commonly occurring in childhood. It is not a venereal or sexually transmitted disease. Although HIV can be transmitted through contaminated needles or blood products, it can also be transmitted through sexual contact. Chlamydia and syphilis are venereal diseases.

37. B: The Truth in Lending Act (TILA) mandates that information regarding the loan must be clearly disclosed to the consumer. It does not dictate the price of fees or interest rates or control who the lender is willing to lend to.

38. D: The Drug Enforcement Agency (DEA) regulates controlled substances such as narcotics and substances that can be used to make illegal drugs. Pseudoephedrine can be used to make methamphetamine. Amoxicillin is a common antibiotic and would be of little interest to the DEA.

39. C: Burns are graded in severity from first to fourth—first being the most mild while fourth-degree burns carrying the highest mortality. Croup is a common respiratory viral illness in children; it is typically not life-threatening. An ankle fracture may be painful but will not kill a person. Conjunctivitis may be a viral, bacterial, or allergic infection of the eye; like ankle fractures they may be uncomfortable but are not life-threatening.

40. D: Hepatitis C is an infection of the liver that is transmitted through sex, infected blood products, or contaminated needles. AIDS is also transmitted through the same mechanisms but dies quickly in the air. A medical provider is much more likely to get hepatitis C from a needle stick than AIDS. Roseola and varicella are viral infections that occur in childhood and are not transmitted through blood.

41. A: Antibiotics hold little interest for the Drug Enforcement Agency (DEA). The DEA controls prescriptive drugs such as benzodiazepines, antipsychotic medications, narcotics, and other medications that have high risk for abuse.

42. C: The Food and Drug Administration (FDA) regulates and supervises the safety, development, and administration of vaccines, medications, and medical supplements. The Centers for Disease Control's (CDC's) job is to identify health risks and devise ways to control or contain potential outbreaks.

43. D: Semen and blood have the highest risk for transmitting AIDS. There is minimal risk of transmitting it through saliva, feces, and urine.

44. A: Implied consent is agreement to something via action without verbally expressing agreement. Rolling up a sleeve for a blood pressure check indicates willingness to have the blood pressure taken.

45. A: An emancipated minor is a person younger than 18 who has been freed from control of his or her parents. He or she must provide for themselves financially, and his or her parents are not legally responsible for the child's actions.

46. B: Medical assistants have a wide breadth of practice that may include administrative duties, documenting vital signs, making patient appointments, administering electrocardiograms, and acting as a patient liaison. Medical assistants cannot prescribe, interpret labs or radiological tests, or perform invasive procedures such as laceration repairs.

47. B: Having capacity means having the cognitive ability to understand medical information being relayed and to make informed, rational decisions based on that information. If a patient's capacity is in question, a psychiatrist is consulted to help make that determination.

48. B: The Food and Drug Administration (FDA) regulates and supervises the safety, development, and administration of vaccines, medications, and medical supplements.

49. B: Subpoena duces tecum is a legal notice that demands a patient must appear in court at a set time and date and provide certain documentation for a case. This may include medical records, bank statements, and computer files. Failure to comply can result in legal penalties such as fines or jail time.

50. C: The physician committed negligence by failing to properly care for the patient. The physician did not notice or did not pay attention to the patient's documented allergies. It may have not been intended, but the physician may face a lawsuit for the error in judgment.

51. D: Generativity versus stagnation generally occurs in the retirement years when people may remain active and involved with community and family. If they fail to do so, they may become isolated and depressed.

52. C: If a patient does not speak English, speaking slowly and loudly will not help him or her understand the message. A translator needs to be present as well as an English-speaking family member. Consent forms written in the patient's native language would also be helpful.

53. A: Acting as a gateway is helpful to a physician when taking messages. The physician may be busy with patients in the office. Getting a brief message from the patient will help the physician triage the importance of the call and help him or her better manage the workload.

54. C: The physician allegedly committed assault. This is a serious crime that can result in fees, loss of licensure, and jail time. To help protect oneself against false claims, a chaperone should always be present.

55. A: Taking the woman's money and keeping it or buying something with it is theft. Depending on the situation and the amount of money taken, it can result in fees, loss of licensure, and jail time. The only appropriate action is to give the woman the correct change.

56. D: Chlamydia is a treatable sexually transmitted disease. She should be advised to use protection with every sexual encounter. She should also be counseled to call prior partners and advise them of her diagnosis, so they can get themselves checked.

57. C: Calling Child Protective Services (CPS) is the most appropriate initial action. Afterward the medical staff should call an orthopedist to evaluate the child's arm. Placing blame on a particular caretaker is unfair and unprofessional. Let CPS investigate the case further.

58. B: A physician may terminate a patient provided that the decision is made in writing and the patient is given appropriate notice to find another physician. Refusing to care for the patient during the notice period is inappropriate.

59. B: Carpeting helps prevent accidents. Its nonslip surface may help prevent against mechanical falls. Dim lighting may help increase the risk of bumping into equipment and falls. Non-adjustable equipment increases the risk of ergonomic injuries. Tile floors can be slick and may increase falls.

60. D: Res ipsa loquitur means that an accident would not have occurred without negligence, for example, if a patient is accidentally given a medication that he or she is allergic to and develops a reaction. Although the incident was an accident, the medical provider was negligent in not reviewing the patient's allergies first.

61. D: Due to privacy laws, a patient's records cannot be released unless authorized by the patient or his or her power of attorney. Checking a person's identification would also be appropriate, but a release still needs to be signed beforehand.

62. C: The medical assistant should report the incident to administration. A mistake was made, and even if there were no negative sequelae from the incident, a safety report should be created.

63. A: The term colo- means colon and the suffix -ostomy means a surgically made opening. A colostomy is where a surgeon reroutes the large intestine through an opening in the abdominal wall. A bag is placed over the opening that collects stool.

64. B: The suffix -itis means inflammation of something. Appendicitis is inflammation of the appendix, cholecystitis is inflammation of the gallbladder, and cystitis is inflammation of the bladder.

65. A: The ulna and the radius are bones located in the forearm, and the olecranon is the medical term for elbow. The tibia and fibula are bones in the lower leg. A phalange can refer to a toe or finger. The humerus is the bone of the upper arm. The femur is the thigh bone. The sternum is the breast plate, which is found in the chest.

66. C: Malleolus is the medical term for ankle. A phalange can refer to a toe or finger. The term for patella means knee. Scapula is the shoulder blade.

67. C: The acetabulum is the socket in the hip where the femur, or thigh bone, joins to the hip. The patella is the medical term for knee, which is below or inferior to the acetabulum. The axilla is the medical term for armpit. The spleen is an organ that helps store red blood cells. It is found in the abdomen. The clavicle or collar bone is superior to, or above, the acetabulum.

68. D: The suffix -acusis refers to hearing. The term hyperacusis means overactive or enhancing hearing ability. The term hyper means excessive. Dysacusis means difficulty hearing. The term dys means disorder or difficulty.

69. C: The prefix a- means without, and the term phasia means speech. Aphasia means without speech. This means that the patient may be unable to form words, unable to understand words, or both. The condition of not being able to do either is known as global aphasia.

70. B: A gynecologist is a specialist in female reproductive disorders. A hematologist is a specialist in disorders of the blood such as sickle cell anemia. A gastroenterologist specializes in digestive anomalies such as reflux. A rheumatologist is a trained specialist in autoimmune disorders of the joints such as rheumatoid arthritis.

71. C: Gloves are standard protection to be used at all times when involved in patient care and the handling of bodily fluids. Protective eyewear, gowns, and masks may be also indicated depending on the situation.

72. A: Office memos are professional documents that are used to announce new protocols, regulations, announcements, or other work-related information. Things such as arguments between staff members should be handled between the involved parties.

73. D: A meniscus is a structure inside of the knee that can be visualized and repaired through an arthroscopy. An arthroscope is an instrument that can visualize structures inside of a joint.

74. B: An inventory is a complete list of supplies and the numbers of each that are currently in the office. This will help keep track of when and how many items need to be replenished.

75. B: The sternum is the medical term for breastplate, which is located in the chest. It helps protect the heart. The clavicle is the collarbone. Scapula is the shoulder blade. An epicondyle is a rounded protuberance of the bone; examples would include knuckles and the lateral and medial epicondyles that flank the elbow.

76. C: Office policy varies, but unpaid bills between 3 to 6 months will typically get sent to a collection agency. A bill that is 3 days late should not have a penalty. A bill that is 3 weeks late may be subject to a late fee. A notice should be sent to the patient regarding the bill's unpaid status. A bill that is 3 years late should obviously have been sent to a collections agency years ago.

77. A: A gastroenterologist specializes in digestive anomalies such as reflux, Crohn's disease, and gastrointestinal neoplasms. Urologists specialize in the genitourinary tract. Orthopedists concentrate on bones and joint. A psychiatrist deals with mental and behavioral disorders.

78. A: The kidneys, liver, stomach, gallbladder, duodenum, and pancreas are structures found in the abdominal cavity. A meniscus is a fibrocartilaginous structure between the femur and tibia in the knee joint. The acetabulum is the socket in the hip where the femur, or thigh bone, joins to the hip. The ureters connect the kidneys to the bladder and are located in the pelvis.

79. C: Petty cash is meant for office-related purchases that may be due to a last-minute need. For example, if there is no more printer paper or manila folders, a staff member may be asked to go out and buy more.

80. C: A dermatologist is a physician who cares for skin disorders such as psoriasis. Cardiologists focus on cardiac disorders and diseases. A psychiatrist deals with mental and behavioral disorders. Urologists specialize in the genitourinary tract.

81. D: Civilian Health and Medical Program of the Department of Veterans Affairs (CHAMPVA) benefits are not granted to those who have been released from service due to misconduct. Their families cannot obtain benefits through the program either. An ex-spouse is eligible for benefits unless he or she remarries. Children and spouses may obtain benefits if their family member is permanently disabled from service-related duty or has died due to complications due to the disability.

82. D: Tricare is a health care program for active military personnel and their spouses, children, and dependents.

83. D: The duodenum is the proximal portion of the small bowel that is found in the abdominal cavity. The trachea, heart, and lungs are all found in the thoracic cavity.

84. C: The spleen is in the left upper quadrant of the abdomen, which is lateral to the liver in the right upper quadrant. The bladder, kidneys, and gallbladder are below or inferior to the liver.

85. A: The sternum, also known as the breastplate, is in front of, or ventral to, the lungs. The trachea is superior or above the lungs. The diaphragm is beneath or inferior to the lungs. The spine is dorsal or in back of the lungs.

86. B: The transverse plane separates body parts into upper and lower portions. The head is separated from the feet by the transverse plane.

87. A: Malleolus is the medical term for ankle. The medical term for thigh bone is the femur. The ankle is inferior to, or below, the femur.

88. A: The adrenal glands are found on top of each kidney. They produce sex hormones and cortisol. The sigmoid colon, appendix, and cervix are inferior to the kidneys.

89. B: The musculoskeletal system includes the bones, muscles, tendons, and ligaments in the body that allow support and movement. Structures such as the ribs and sternum protect important organs such as the heart and lungs.

90. C: The chain comprises of six sequential stages. If any of the links in the chain are missing, then an infectious disease is unlikely to be transmitted. There is the causative agent, whether it is bacteria, fungi, virus, prior, and so on. Then there is the source or reservoir in which the pathogen proliferates. Third is the exit route, or how the pathogen escapes its host. Next is the mode of transmission. Some pathogens may be transmitted through blood, whereas others may be transmitted through droplets or a fecal-oral route. The following step is the mode of entry into the next host, which is similar to the exit route. Last is the susceptible host.

91. C: Immunocompromised patients would be ideal susceptible hosts. Immunocompromised patients such as those with AIDS, cancer, or chronic illness are susceptible hosts because their immune systems are either poorly functioning or nonfunctional, making it easy for infection to spread.

92. D: Pyelonephritis is an infection of the kidneys caused by an ascending kidney infection. The genitourinary system is affected. It usually fully resolves with a course of antibiotics.

93. D: A parasite is a pathogen that needs a host cell to proliferate and survive. It derives energy and nutrients from its host. An example of a parasite is a tapeworm.

94. A: Bacteria have cell walls. Viruses have a unique protein coat. The protein coat is also called a capsid, which contains the genetic information of the virus.

95. B: If a mistake is made while writing a note, make a single line through the error, write error, and initial and time the correction. It is illegal to use whiteout or erase a medical chart. Throwing out the entire note and starting over isn't necessary.

96. B: The mammary glands or breasts are in front of, or ventral to, the spine. In contrast, the spine is dorsal to, or in back of, the breasts.

97. B: A normal heart rate in an adult human is 60 to 100 beats per minute. Those who are elderly, in excellent physical condition, or sleeping may have lower heart rates. Conditions such as stress, exercise, thyroid dysfunctions, or illness may cause an elevated heart rate.

98. D: The appendix is an accessory organ found at the ileocecal junction. Nonpregnant patients with normal anatomy will typically have pain in the right lower quadrant of the abdomen.

99. A: A pulse oximeter is a medical device that indirectly monitors the oxygen saturation of a patient's blood. A normal reading should be 94 to 100 percent. Patients with chronic obstructive pulmonary disease or pneumonia may have lower readings. A pulse ox of 75 percent would require intubation and mechanical ventilation. A pulse ox of 50 percent is not consistent with life.

100. A: Leukemia is a type of malignancy of the bone marrow and blood that affects the hematologic system.

101. C: There are three portals of entry for an infection to spread: ingestion (fecal-oral transmission), inhalation (respiratory droplet), and penetration (sexually transmitted disease). Infections are not transmitted through sweating.

102. B: A pulse oximeter is a medical device that indirectly monitors the oxygen saturation of a patient's blood. It is usually placed on a peripheral body part. The fingertip is most commonly used but can also be placed on a toe or an earlobe.

103. C: The normal average body temperature in humans is 98.6 degrees Fahrenheit or 37 degrees Celsius.

104. C: One of the most common and easiest spots to palpate a pulse is the radial artery. This can be felt on the ventral aspect of the wrist. The popliteal artery is much more difficult to palpate because it's located behind the knee. The femoral artery is found in the groin, which may be awkward to palpate during a routine office visit. The dorsalis pedis pulse is located on top of the foot. It can be used to palpate a pulse, but the wrist is generally more easily accessible.

105. B: Celiac disease is an autoimmune disorder causing inflammation and damage to the small intestine when patients ingest gluten products.

106. A: The chief complaint section should be a few words that summarize why the patient is in the hospital or clinic. Habits such as drug or alcohol use or type of employment belong in the social history. Precipitating or alleviating factors belong in the history of present illness section.

107. D: Fungi are eukaryotic organisms that are commonly found in mold or yeast. Mushrooms are a type of fungi.

108. B: A reservoir refers to where a pathogen lives and proliferates. Soil, blood, semen, and mold are some examples of reservoirs.

109. A: Instrumentation used for a colonoscopy should be sterilized after every use. They are used to examine patients' rectums and large bowels, which are contaminated and cannot be cleaned using ordinary methods.

110: C. Endometriosis is a condition where uterine tissue is deposited throughout various sites in the body. The condition may be asymptomatic, or it may cause painful sexual intercourse, dysmenorrhea, menorrhagia, and infertility.

111. D: A patient is prone when he or she is lying facedown. A patient who is lying on his or her side is in the lateral recumbent position. The Trendelenburg position is where the patient is lying supine with the feet higher than the head by about 30 degrees. They are in the supine position when lying flat on their back.

112. C: Most patients should get their first colonoscopy at 50 years of age. If they have a certain condition that predisposes them to colorectal cancer, then they should obtain one earlier. If they have a first-degree relative with colorectal cancer, then they should be screened 10 years earlier than their family member's initial diagnosis. So, if a patient has a sister diagnosed with colorectal cancer at 46, then the patient should get his or her first colonoscopy when he or she is 36.

113. C: It is recommended that women should perform self breast exams every month, usually after their period. Menses can cause growth of fibroadenomas and fibrocystic breast disease due to changing hormones. Therefore, it is recommended to do it after the menses has ended to prevent unnecessary false alarms.

114. A: The Trendelenburg position is where the patient is lying supine with the feet higher than the head by about 30 degrees. Reverse Trendelenburg is where the head is higher than the feet by about 30 degrees. Fowlers position is where the patient is sitting upright with knees slightly bent. Lithotomy position is where the patient is supine with knees bent and spread apart; it is commonly used when doing gynecological procedures or exams.

115. D: A patient with hypertension should limit his or her sodium intake. Excess sodium causes retention of water, which raises blood pressure.

116. D: The international normalized ratio (INR) measures the viscosity of blood. It is used to help monitor treatment in patients taking blood thinners like Coumadin.

117. A: BUN and creatinine are lab markers that monitor kidney function. They may become elevated when a patient is dehydrated, is severely ill (such as sepsis), or is taking certain medications that may affect the kidneys.

118. B: Celiac disease is an autoimmune disorder causing inflammation and damage to the small intestine when patients ingest gluten products. Products such as wheat, barley, and rye contain gluten. These are common ingredients in bread, crackers, and cakes.

119. C: H. pylori is a type of bacteria that frequently causes chronic gastritis and ulcers. It increases the risk of stomach cancer as well.

120. B: Patients who are lactose intolerant do not have the enzyme lactase to help digest dairy products, causing flatulence and abdominal discomfort. Yogurt, milk, ice cream, and cheeses should be limited or avoided.

121. C: Items such as drug and alcohol use, exercise, and occupation belong in the social history.

122. C: A blood pressure should be taken once a patient has been seated or lying down for several minutes. If it is taken after an activity, it may be falsely elevated.

123. B: A normal respiratory rate in a healthy adult ranges between 12 and 20 breaths per minute. Below this range is called bradypnea, and above this range is called tachypnea.

124. B: Skin glue should never be used during a suture removal. Suture removals usually take place 5 to 10 days after being placed. Open wounds should not be closed 24 hours after the initial injury.

After this point the wound has become colonized with bacteria, and closing it significantly increases the risk of infection.

125. A: Making gradually enlarging circles during skin prep prevents from contaminating a previously prepped site.

126. D: Insulin is usually administered as a subcutaneous injection. In cased of severe hyperglycemia, it is administered as a continuous intravenous infusion.

127. B: Those with very poorly controlled diabetics should be advised to check their blood sugars three times a day before meals and before bedtime. They should make a log of their results along with what they've eaten and bring it to their physician for review.

128. B: Tobacco smoke predisposes people to many things such as heart attacks (myocardial infarctions), chronic lung diseases like asthma and bronchitis, and malignancies like lung cancer. Diabetes is not a direct complication of tobacco abuse.

129. C: The influenza vaccine is an intramuscular injection, although it can also be inhaled. It is recommended that patients get them every year if they have no allergies or contraindications.

130. C: Once a woman becomes 18 or becomes sexually active (whichever comes first), she should get Pap smears every year to screen for cervical cancer.

131. D: The pneumococcal vaccine is a live vaccine and cannot be administered to those who are immunocompromised. A patient with diabetes may be more prone to certain minor infections such as urinary tract infections but is not considered immunocompromised.

132. B: A greenstick fracture involves a bend in the bone on one side and a small, incomplete break on the contralateral cortex. This type of fracture is commonly seen in children, whose bones are softer than adults.

133. A: Ischemic strokes are the most common. Approximately 80 percent of strokes that occur are ischemic, whereas the remainder is hemorrhagic.

134. D: Antibiotics are used for bacterial infections and play no role in the initial treatment of poisoning.

135. A: Absence seizures are typically seen in young children and involve blank staring episodes associated with amnesia about the event. It may be misdiagnosed as attention deficit disorder.

136. A: Diabetic ketoacidosis is a serious condition with incredibly high levels of ketones and blood glucose. The treatment includes insulin, IV fluids, and correction of electrolyte abnormalities.

137. A: An oblique fracture is a diagonal break in the bone. A dislocation is where the bone comes out of its joint. A transverse fracture is a horizontal fracture. A comminuted fracture is where the bone splinters off into several pieces.

138. A: There are two halves of the brain that control the contralateral aspects of the body. When a person has a right-sided stroke, the left side will be affected.

139. A: An X-ray is a test that evaluates bones and joints. It is the best initial test to examine bony injuries.

140. C: Syncope is the medical term for passing out. There are many etiologies that may cause syncope, such as stress, hemorrhage, hypoglycemia, bradycardia, pregnancy, vertigo, stroke, and hypoxia.

141. D: Ataxia is the presence of an abnormal gait. This may be due to visual disturbances, stroke, neurologic malignancies or abnormalities, or certain diseases such as Creutzfeldt-Jakob disease.

142. B: Wheezing is an abnormal lung sound caused by narrowed airways. This can be seen in patients with chronic lung diseases such as chronic obstructive pulmonary disease (COPD) or asthma or with acute infections such as pneumonia. Nebulizer treatments and steroids are the mainstays of therapy.

143. D: Per advanced cardiac life support (ACLS) protocol, pulseless ventricular fibrillation and pulseless ventricular tachycardia are the only rhythms that are shockable arrhythmias.

144. A: Grand mal seizures are classic seizures that involve loss of consciousness, drooling, and generalized body tremors. Because other types of seizures may also involve drooling, A is the best answer.

145. C: If there is any question with the seal on the bottle, the expiration date, or the contents, the vaccine should be safely discarded.

146. C: Focal tremors are signs of simple partial seizures. It usually involves a single extremity (although may include both extremities on the ipsilateral side) and does not include loss of consciousness.

147. B: The six rights of medication administration are aimed at preventing errors involving medication. These include right patient, right medication, right dose, right route, right time, and right documentation.

148. D: Diabetes insipidus is a serious condition that results in abnormal excessive urination resulting in excessive thirst and electrolyte abnormalities. It may be caused by brain damage or malignancy, mental illness (iatrogenic), and pregnancy. It is not related to hemorrhage.

149. B: A normal respiratory rate in a healthy adult ranges between 12 and 20 breaths per minute. Below this range is called bradypnea, and above this range is called tachypnea.

150. A: A sublingual medication is placed underneath the tongue and absorbed through the oral mucosa. The oral mucosa is rich in vasculature, and the medication can be absorbed into the blood quickly.

151. A: There are many items found in the crash cart, including sterile gowns and gloves, certain medications, and items used for intubation such as laryngoscopes, syringes, needles, and alcohol swabs. Stethoscopes are not typically found in crash cards as medical professionals carry their own.

152. D: Itching, hives, and nausea are uncomfortable, but the most feared drug reaction involves anaphylaxis. Anaphylaxis may occur instantaneously or after several minutes or hours. It involves mild symptoms progressing to more severe systemic symptoms such as facial swelling, difficulty breathing, airway edema, and hypotension due to vasodilation. Epinephrine, Benadryl, IV fluids, steroids, and sometimes intubation are needed.

153. C: According to advanced cardiac life support (ACLS) and basic life support (BLS) protocols, the examiner should tap the chest of a seemingly unresponsive patient and ask if he or she is awake.

If there is no response, call for help, have someone get a defibrillator (if possible), check a pulse, and start chest compressions if none can be found.

154. B: Rabies is a concern with feral animal bites. The most common causes of rabies include foxes, raccoons, skunks, and bats. Prophylactic treatment is given in the form of serial injections over the course of a few weeks.

155. B: Per ACLS protocol, a provider should administer about 100 quality chest compressions per minute to provide the patient with the best chance of survival.

156. B: A peripheral pulse found in the arm or leg should never be used during a resuscitation effort. If the blood pressure is low, a faint pulse may not be able to be palpated. An easily accessible central pulse should be used, such as the femoral artery or preferably the carotid artery.

157. C: Vertigo is a condition that involves nausea, vomiting, dizziness, and ataxia due to an inner ear dysfunction. Seizures are not a common sign of this disorder.

158. D: The Heimlich maneuver is performed on a conscious patient who is choking. Once he or she loses consciousness, the Heimlich maneuver should be discontinued, and basic life support (BLS) should be performed until paramedics arrive.

159. D: There are six pregnancy categories: A, B, C, D, N, and X. Pregnancy category A means that the drug is safe to take in pregnancy due to extensive animal and human studies. Pregnancy category B means that there are no studies that have shown definite risk to the fetus. Pregnancy category C means that risk to the fetus has not been ruled out. Pregnancy category D means that studies have shown risk to the fetus, but the medication may be worth the risk due to benefit to the mother. An example would be chemotherapy agents. Pregnancy category X means that there are significant fetal deformities that will occur and the medication is contraindicated in pregnant women. Pregnancy category N means that the Food and Drug Administration hasn't classified the medication yet.

160. D: Anyone who has taken a basic life support (BLS) course can do cardiopulmonary resuscitation (CPR). The BLS course involves a written examination and a simulation of maneuvers performed on a mannequin.

161. C: A scratch test involves scratching the superficial layer of the skin and introducing potential allergies to the area. If a reaction occurs, then the patient is allergic to that particular substance.

162. B: Beta human chorionic gonadotropin (beta hcg) is produced by the developing embryo. The level in most normal pregnancies doubles every 48 to 72 hours in the first 4 weeks of pregnancy. After that point it generally increases every 72 to 96 hours. Eventually the hormone levels off later on in the pregnancy. Because her hcg didn't quite double, there is no way to determine at this point if the pregnancy is viable.

163. A: Erythrocyte sedimentation rate (ESR) and c-reactive protein (CRP) are nonspecific markers of inflammation that can be seen with infections, acute pathology such as a heart attack, or stress.

164. C: Epstein-Barr virus (EBV) causes mononucleosis, aka mononucleosis, or mono. Mono is respiratory illness generally seen in young adults that presents with fatigue, anorexia, pharyngitis, and abdominal pain. It generally resolves on its own without complication.

165. B: Platelets or thrombocytes aid in clotting. They stick together to form a plug at the site of injury to prevent excessive bleeding. Severe thrombocytopenia may cause spontaneous and excessive bleeding.

166. A: The scratch test is one of the more common dermal allergy tests, but another test involves injecting a small amount of the allergen into the superficial layers of the skin.

167. D: Calibration means to adjust the measurement of a device to ensure the most accurate results.

168. B: A fixative may be applied to stabilize or preserve something to use it later. Skin scrapings may be saved with a fixative to prevent cell death, so they can be examined by a microscope later.

169. C: The corpus callosum is the thick band of nerve fibers that separates the right and left sides of the brain. It facilitates communication between the two sides.

170. C: Pure tone audiometry helps detect hearing threshold levels and determine the type of hearing loss that has occurred. Weber and Rinne tests use a tuning fork to help determine which ear has suffers the loss and if it is a conductive or sensory loss. The cold caloric test is used to assess brain damage in comatose patients.

171. C: To obtain a 12-lead ECG, a total of 10 electrodes are used. Six precordial chest leads and four limb leads are used.

172. C: A Holter monitor is worn for 24 to 48 hours to help evaluate for the presence of arrhythmias. In the event that a significant arrhythmia is detected, a pacemaker may need to be placed. It cannot evaluate the structures of the heart.

173. C: Atrial fibrillation is the abnormal arrhythmia where the atria do not rhythmically contract. This can cause palpitations, chest pain, dizziness, and syncope. It can result in pulmonary emboli, heart attack, and stroke. On an ECG the p-waves are irregular and not associated with QRS complexes.

174. D: The sinoatrial (SA) node is the heart's natural pacemaker. If it fails, the atrioventricular (AV) node will act as backup albeit at a slower pace than a normal heart rate.

175. A: A normal QRS is 0.08 to 0.012 seconds or two to three small boxes on an ECG.

176. C: Endocarditis, or the presence of vegetation(s) on a heart valve, can be diagnosed with direct visualization on a transthoracic echo or a transesophageal echo. An ECG is not a diagnostic test for endocarditis.

177. D: A normal PR interval is 0.012 to 0.20 seconds on an ECG. Anything longer than 0.20 seconds is called a prolonged interval. Fixed, prolonged PR intervals are seen in first-degree heart block.

178. D: A Jaeger card is used to assess visual acuity. It has a large single letter at the top, with each successive line increasing in number of letters and decreasing in size.

179. B: Glaucoma involves the presence of increased intraocular pressure. It is caused by overproduction of aqueous humor (fluid) and decreased outflow of the fluid. If left untreated it can lead to blindness.

180. A: A normal PR interval is 0.012 to 0.20 seconds on an ECG. Anything longer than 0.20 seconds is called a prolonged interval. Fixed, prolonged PR intervals are seen in first-degree heart block.

Thank You

We at Mometrix would like to extend our heartfelt thanks to you, our friend and patron, for allowing us to play a part in your journey. It is a privilege to serve people from all walks of life who are unified in their commitment to building the best future they can for themselves.

The preparation you devote to these important testing milestones may be the most valuable educational opportunity you have for making a real difference in your life. We encourage you to put your heart into it—that feeling of succeeding, overcoming, and yes, conquering will be well worth the hours you've invested.

We want to hear your story, your struggles and your successes, and if you see any opportunities for us to improve our materials so we can help others even more effectively in the future, please share that with us as well. **The team at Mometrix would be absolutely thrilled to hear from you!** So please, send us an email (support@mometrix.com) and let's stay in touch.

If you feel as though you need additional help, please check out the other resources we offer:

Study Guide:
http://MometrixStudyGuides.com/MedicalAssistant

Flashcards: http://MometrixFlashcards.com/MedicalAssistant